Tanzanian Women in Their Own Words

Tanzanian Women in Their Own Words

Stories of Disability and Illness

Sheryl Feinstein and Nicole C. D'Errico

LEXINGTON BOOKS

A division of

ROWMAN & LITTLEFIELD PUBLISHERS, INC.
Lanham • Boulder • New York • Toronto • Plymouth, UK

Published by Lexington Books
A division of Rowman & Littlefield Publishers, Inc.
A wholly owned subsidiary of The Rowman & Littlefield Publishing Group, Inc.
4501 Forbes Boulevard, Suite 200, Lanham, Maryland 20706
http://www.lexingtonbooks.com

Estover Road
Plymouth PL6 7PY
United Kingdom

British Library Cataloguing in Publication Information Available

Library of Congress Cataloging-in-Publication Data

Feinstein, Sheryl.
  Tanzanian women in their own words : stories of disability and illness / Sheryl
Feinstein and Nicole C. D'Errico.
    p. cm.
  Includes bibliographical references and index.
  ISBN 978-0-7391-4056-7 (cloth : alk. paper) — ISBN 978-0-7391-4057-4 (pbk. : alk.
paper) — ISBN 978-0-7391-4058-1 (electronic)
   1. Women with disabilities—Health and hygiene—Tanzania—Anecdotes.
2. Women—Health and hygiene—Tanzania—Anecdotes. 3. Health services
accessibility—Tanzania—Anecdotes. 4. Women—Tanzania—Social conditions—
Anecdotes. I. D'Errico, Nicole C. II. Title.
RA564.88.F45 2010
362.108209678—dc22   2009032407

Printed in the United States of America

Dedication

To my mother, Kathleen,
whose life—
mediated by her mother's illness and
abridged by her own—
was a work of art.
N.C. D.

To my grandson, Joe,
who brings me joy—
may these stories inspire you.
S.F.

Contents

Acknowledgments

This book exists wholly because of the brave spirits of the women who shared their stories. Their smiles, sobs, lessons, and fierce strengths remain as invaluable gifts on the shelves of our hearts. Their suffering and their triumphs gave birth to this book.

Thank you to the faculty and staff at Tumaini University, DIRA ELCT, Anglican Mission, and Neema Craft. Their generosity in arranging, facilitating and coordinating introductions, transportation, meeting places, and interpreters was essential in bringing this project to fruition.

S. F. & N. C. D.

To my unrelentingly brilliant mentors past—June Foley, Brad Lewis—and present—Alyson Young, Lançe Gravlee and Russ Bernard—whose profound influence on me makes me want to list their names as authors of this book."Past" and "present" demarcate chronology, for my advisors' roles have been (and I pray will remain) tireless and enduring. My gratitude to this group of people grows every day. To Mary Marshall Clark, who brought me to Oral History as if it was a sandbox, encouraging me to jump in and play. To my Mother of the Heart, Felice Kaufmann, who is my How-To guide for life. To David Cohen, who makes my hills less steep, and whose inner strength is the net which never fails to break my fall.

To my grandmother, Rose D'Errico, who, like the women in this book, manages to grow as a person when the world is most frightening. To Ron and Marie Antonelli, who constantly remind me what is good in the world, mostly recently with Eve. To Marie, specifically, who is the glue between the fragments. To my father, Frank D'Errico, whose words of encouragement *never take a back seat to anyone,* continue to inspire me, day in, day out. His endless support and unwavering commitment to fatherhood, make me wonder what the world would look like if every child grew up in the shadow of his love.

And finally, to Scott Feinstein, who, by no small measure, is responsible for the existence of this book.

N.C. D.

To Scott and James Feinstein, Jen and Chris Sharp, Susan Gibbons, Jack and Phyllis Gibbons and Vicki Bachmayer, whose long distance support, humor and encouragement helped me find harmony in the reality of my life. To Sophia Sabrow and Lisa Hecht who shared my experience in Tanzania and whose on-site support made me smile and expanded my horizons. To the U.S. Fulbright Scholars Program for offering me the opportunity to spend a year in Tanzania getting to know its generous and engaging people. To Belinda Kaffar at Augustana College who always encourages my work and lightens my load. And particularly to Rachel Feinstein whose visit to Tanzania brought me joy and comfort.

S. F.

A portion of the proceeds from this book will be donated to communities in Tanzania to benefit the needs and medical issues of women.

Introduction

I feel bad, day and night you can see me in tears. I cry for months. I beg my sisters to bring me poison, I want to die.

—Faustina, *reflecting on her accident*

Then that afternoon my sister comes to me and she pretend she open something to give me. She says, "Faustina I have brought the poison, do you want it? Now you have started a new life." A beautiful life, I had reason to live.

—Faustina, *later in the interview, recalling*
the birth of her daughter

The stories written within the pages of this book—the lives into which our interviews provide a window—are remarkable stories of human suffering. During our research in Tanzania, interview after interview caused us to reflect on the nature of suffering and triumphs, and on the capacity to make meaning of the experiences life presents to us. Each oral history interview we were graciously granted brought us along with the brave women who were reflecting on their lives—reflecting on the challenges, reflecting on the joys. At the end of every long day of research, we felt as though our souls had experienced something truly profound—the byproduct of the osmosis occurring in front of our eyes, as we lived and re-lived the women's lives with them. We could not hold the stories in. We could not allow them to remain as scribbled words in a pile of field notes, as magnetic variations on the wound-up tape within our cassettes. *The stories needed to be shared.*

Unlike the women whose voices we transcribed, we knew our lives gave us the kind of privilege needed to make these words public. This book attempts to accomplish the weighty task we found ourselves carrying, as the receptors of the stories, the morals, *the meanings* the women wove with their words into quilts of life. It is our hope that these stories move you as they moved us, that they render you an active participant in a dialogue with the world, with the women in our book, and with your own life.

Tanzanian Women in Their Own Words: Stories of Disability and Illness consists of fourteen chapters focusing on common health issues faced by women in Tanzania. Each chapter begins with an introduction which paints a picture of the location and circumstances of the individual being interviewed and gives general background information. Every woman then tells her own life story, in first person perspective, allowing the reader to intimately engage with the storyteller. Their stories are followed by a conclusion and discussion questions which, by placing the narratives in a greater cultural context, challenges readers to consider how they would write their own narratives, to think about the cultural context in which they would place *their* stories.

In his reflections on listening to the stories of those in the developing world in grave medical crisis, James Orbinski wrote: "Speaking is the first political act. It is the first act of liberty, and it always implicitly involves another. In speaking, one recognizes 'I am and I am not alone.'" We hope you enjoy reading and experiencing these stories. In doing so, you too become complicit in this first political act. You too are recognizing the necessity in telling those who feel they might be alone, that they are not. Together, we enter the second act.

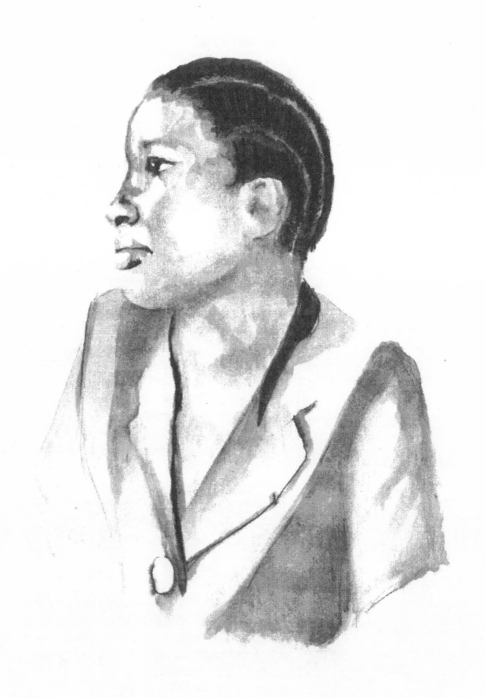

Chapter 1

Atu

We gathered at Atu's home. It stands in deep contrast to other homes in the village, which are made of mud; Atu's home is made from cement, a sign of affluence. Her home is owned by the health center where she works and reflects her comfortable lifestyle. She has two sofas and large, color photos on the wall. An empty box that held drinking glasses, a remnant of a treasured gift from Germany, is proudly displayed.

Atu is a nurse in a remote village in the Iringa Region. She is a proud and determined woman who curiously blends self-assuredness with self-consciousness. She is of small stature, an unassuming woman. As she turns toward you, one cannot help but be disturbed by her face. One side is lovely, with soft, appealing features; the other side has been mutilated. Her eye bulges out, her chin juts at a wrong angle, and her cheek is drawn dramatically in as scars traverse the contours of her face. As she speaks it is clear that she is aware of her facial disfiguration and its affect on how she will be received. She offers us tea and then begins to talk; she is articulate as she tells her story. Within minutes, the marks on her face are forgotten.

ATU

My name is Atu; it means "God Saves Us." I was born in Iringa Region in Ipagora in 1971, I am 36 years old. I'm from the Nyakyusa tribe from Mebea in the southwestern part of the country. Like all tribes in Africa, there are things that are unique to my tribe. We have a tribal language and we learn to speak KiSwahili, because of this we can talk to other tribes.

3

In my tribe females never live together with boys; when a girl marries the boy, she isn't to be seen by the father-in-law. For instance, if I married I would never see my husband's father—it's a tradition. We have traditional ethics. We mainly marry in tribe. If someone marries outside their tribe others call them bad names.

In the Nyakyusa tribe it is a shame to see you in menses—don't mention it, it's a secret. Girls tell their mom or parents. They don't do circumcision in my tribe, male or female. If mom is in labor pain she is isolated. These things are not talked about.

When someone dies, a grave is dug right outside the house. They plant banana trees on top of graves, it's a tradition. They do some witchcraft. Grandparents worshipped things that were godless; worshipped ghosts. Others are witches. If they don't want someone to have good things, they put a curse on them. This is my tribe.

Both my mom and dad were Nyakyusa, but from different villages. Nitwele is my mom; she is 47 years old now and lives in Ipagora. My dad died three years ago, he was 67. My father didn't have other wives—my parents were saved, they knew God. Even Christians have many wives. You need fear. My family is Christian.

I was the third born of five alive. I have three brothers and one sister—all are alive. We were eight, but three passed. Two brothers and one sister died. First boy that died, Mussa, was in Form 2 secondary boarding schooling at 15. I don't know why he died, could be food. When kids are in boarding school there is not much caring, many get sick, bad food, bad water. Enocki, another brother, was 20 when he died in 2002. He had no family, it was a car accident. He was living in Isimila. Neema, my sister, was 26 years old when she died in an accident. She had one baby girl. The baby lives in Ipagora with my mother. Here when a mother dies a man gets another wife and sometimes that mom doesn't love the child, so better for the child to go to the grandma. That is what happened to my sister's baby. Many children live with their grandma in our country.

My parents were farmers. In the beginning my father was working in Ipagora, then he moved to Isimila. But when my father died the family moved back to Ipagora. As a teenager I started working in the field with my brothers and sister. When my father was alive we all worked in the field, we sold maize. We had food and shelter, life was good. Our parents were examples to us.

I attended school—primary, secondary, and nursing school. My older brothers do not have as much education. When my father was working we had a lot of money so my brothers thought—why go to school, we have money. My father always mentioned to me to go to school. My father went to Standard 4 in primary school, he quit because his father died young.

My father was very gentle. My mom was also gentle. She loves all the family. Their parents were gentle too, they loved them. Brothers and sisters are all gentle. When life is hard you see if the family is good to you or not. When my father died things became hard, but my family was good.

A tumor is what is wrong with my face. When I was first sick—just a small tumor—I was schooling, I told doctor in nursing school, asked them to remove it. First time tumor was removed I was 29 and I had two more years of school. Doctors wanted to do surgery right away; some others were waiting six months for a surgery. I said wait till I go on holiday and tell mom and dad. School paid for the first surgery. Even after operation there was no pain, only last time there was pain because of feeding tubes for three weeks. It's been removed more than eight times, last year it was huge.

Second surgery was in 2001. Doctors were very loving—doctors do a very good job, but I had to pay a lot of money—50,000 tsh [$50.00], but once I agreed, the doctor said if I want him to remove it I must pay more money—there is much corruption in my country. I had more surgeries, one in 2004, it cost 200,000 tsh ($200), money came from father and Anglican Diocese. In 2006 the Diocese family helped. There have now been eight to ten surgeries, many times just a week recovery for the surgery. I plan to have another surgery soon; the tumor is growing inside my mouth.

I found out another problem with the tumor. I first went to Kehesa, then went to Iringa, they said it was cancer and sent me to Mbabilia. I had treatment, but it wasn't cancer. I was relieved. In 2000, doctors did a biopsy and told me it was a certain type of tumor and there was a high chance it would reoccur. When I went to Dar again in 2005 they agreed it was this type of tumor. Then in 2006 went to Mbabilia, I went to two more doctors to investigate and got same results. 2006 was last surgery. Still have a hard chin, but it is reduced.

Dar es Salaam, this is where the last surgery was. I was there four weeks. I don't know if they got it all. I was totally out from 2:00 am to 6:00 am. I knew nothing; I was in ICU all night. There was great pain. They were very humble to me, they showed love. The medical staff respected me more because I was in nursing. Villager would be treated the same, but they would not have as good a room, we have rooms for staff.

My mother, brother, and sister-in-law came to Dar es Salaam for the last surgery. My brother and his wife stayed two weeks. They always phone me, "Oh, how are you?" They showed they cared. My mom was always crying. She did not cry because she was worried, she cried because she could not accept that I was sick and that my face was damaged.

I feel bad, having surgery on my face. I had some dreams that I wanted to have a family and have a husband. But now . . . (sad pause) I am thankful I have my health. I feel bad about not getting married, because if I would get married I don't need to buy things because at my wedding there are lots of gifts. If you do not marry there are no gifts.

I was sad, only God helped me be at peace. I was angry, said, "Why me God?" for months. But family, friends, and doctors encouraged me. My mom worried I wouldn't be able to care for her. Mom said, "Atu care for me." I must always give her money, she always asks and I have known she needs it. After the tumor I thought, now it's Atu, I have to make my own life. It was empowering.

I wanted to have higher education, have my own house, to have a family which has an education. But now when I get the money I save for my health. And if I want more learning, need more money. I expected my father would contribute to me, but no more. When I get money I have to save for my face and my mother needs money. Here in Tanzania mothers rely on their daughter for everything. Boy looks after his family. But some don't care to save their parents, but I wanted to. My elders had no education. Mom says if anything wrong with her she goes to live with Atu (said this with pride, and lightly patted her chest). My own child needs money to go to school.

If I had a husband I would have two or three kids. The dream of getting married is done — to some men it might be a burden to him. If I was married I would stay with him forever and take care of him, but men leave if burdened. It would hurt me too much to be abandoned.

I wanted a daughter and now I have Bertha. Somebody in Dar is father of Bertha. Didn't love him, just wanted a baby. I knew what I had to do. My parents were sad when they found I was pregnant. They didn't know I was planning this. I called them and apologized. I was afraid of what they would do. My father prayed and accepted me. My sister had got pregnant before and my parents chased her away. I think I presented it different to them. I explained my condition, they agreed with me, they understood. That is love. [She tears up, speaking of her parent's kindness.]

I was nine months along and nobody knew; I went to the Bishop to apologize for getting pregnant and say I leave now to have the baby. Bishop didn't believe me; he thought I could not be having a baby. He said, "Did you tell your parents?" I said yes. He said, "Do you want to rest now before you have the baby?" I said yes. At first the Diocese couldn't understand why I got pregnant, but now they know why.

I knew I had done very bad mistake to my parents and job and I needed to take care of myself or they would think I had an abortion. If I lost the baby all would think I aborted. So I went to all to apologize. I stayed home for three weeks and rested and then gave birth. I went home to Isimila for birth, stayed at home for one year after that.

It was a very nice birth. I was schooling to be a midwife so it was practical with me. Water had ruptured, membrane, no pain. I was cutting vegetables at home and my water broke. At 3:00 pm I went to the hospital and at 11:00 pm doctors examined me and said "Give her pitocin and at 8:00 am if no progress, call me, maybe have a C-section." I had edema, I was very swollen, uncomfortable. Pitocin is very, very bad, contractions very bad. Many pregnant women in a room, it was crowded, and women screamed. One woman screams, "I will die, I will die." Some women walk the floors, stopping for contractions; others lie in bed. No one gets pain medicine. We suffer alone. My mother, sister, and sister-in-law are not in the room with me, but they are in the hospital. The hospital not let them in my room. When time to deliver, the doctor and nurse move me to a room for two or three people. Two others are pushing in the room. I lie on plastic mattresses, the pain is very bad. Pushing was very fine. 11:05 am I gave birth. Birth painful, but I have my baby. I am someone's mother.

It was very nice to see the baby. The doctor took the baby and wrapped her in a blanket to keep her warm. He placed her under warm lamp. I scrubbed my birthing bed and moved myself back to other room where mothers in labor. I breastfed her that day and I continued to for 1½ years. Many breastfeed longer. I stopped because I had to travel to Dar es Salaam for another surgery. Left baby with father and my mom went with me.

Her dad, Bertha's, doesn't care anything about her, nothing. Never came to see the baby and I don't care. Maybe at first I cared. I couldn't understand why a dad would not want to see such a beautiful baby. But now I know; I want my baby to have a peaceful life. With her dad, there may be no peace. If it's sad about our situation, people should be sad for me, not the baby. Bertha is well, I am fine raising Bertha.

I finished nursing school in 2002. Muhanbingeto was where I lived when Bertha was born. I had been working with AIDS patients for two years. Now I was in Ipagora with my family. The year I stayed at home was fine; everyone loved Bertha. I left job when I was pregnant and then they called me to return to work. My contract was for four years because they were my sponsors. I worked two years, took leave for baby, and then went back. Now the contract is done and I have a job with the Anglican Diocese. I like working for the Diocese because it is peaceful. Government hospitals pay much more. Hope to talk to Diocese about paying more. I have a secret to tell you—sometimes I'm not paid at work. I haven't been paid in three months. No money for me, my daughter, my mom. When my father was alive they would give us food.

I moved to this village with the Diocese. In this village there is interaction between the tribes—Gogo marry Hehe and Maasai—we are all relatives. Our problems are ours, we accept them. And we accept each other. Most people are illiterate, very hard to work with the people I do here. I like to serve. I also like to cultivate; here they grow rice and a good harvest. I have a business and it gives me extra money.

I don't think people see me differently because of my face, because they want to have Atu give them injection to get well [this is said with great pride]. Maybe kids don't like me, afraid of my face, but I don't care. People don't treat you differently; even if not educated they treat you fine because they know I will help. I became a nurse because I like to serve people, it's in my heart and blood. When I see someone come to the hospital and they can't walk and they leave walking it . . . [pats her heart]. I am proud to be here in the village. You gain much experience. In a big hospital only do what doctors say, they don't know they need to change mother's position during labor. Here I can do anything, although I become tired. Even with no doctor I can attend the patient.

I don't think of having more children, but think of adopting; money is a problem. If I have another child, I will adopt. I'm still thinking of doing it. There's a center where they keep orphans. Some people throw them away there. Only one, I want one baby, I want a boy. I have a girl.

Yes, I think seriously about it, maybe after two years. I plan to start building a house this year, and next year Bertha must start school. I want to send Bertha to a better school than what is in the village, she should have gone to school this year, but I waited. I did not want her to leave me. I will send her to school in Ipagora, a bigger town and my mother lives there. Only problem now is money. If I had money I would do it now.

That is my life, now I will tell about my job. It is hard work. There is diarrhea, scurvy wherever you move, but here so much malaria. Before I came here I was very worried; this area has much malaria—worried about my child. Very different weather—very hot, mosquitoes like it. There is a big outbreak of malaria in rainy season and all year long. I treat many diseases: pneumonia, acute staph infections, eye infections, nutrition disorders, skin infection, minor wounds, worm manifestations. Those with malaria and anemia die the most. When patient comes to me and says neck aches, I take body temperature; if it's hot I think it might be malaria and give her drugs.

Giving birth is very difficult in village, I know many sad stories. Moms aren't emotionally prepared for birth; don't come to the clinic till ready to give birth, so they know nothing. I feel very bad. There is very high local belief that older moms must have traditional birth at home. Last week a woman gave birth at home with a traditional healer; the placenta would not come out. She almost died; we got her to hospital in Iringa. Now she is home.

They give birth at home with traditional healers, or, on the way here! Moms walk many kilometers to reach our health center while they are in labor. They carry two buckets while they walk, one filled with water to wash their new baby and to clean the area and the other to put their placenta in. Sometimes other women accompany them to the health center and help them carry the buckets. Many women grow tired or are far in labor while they walk. They give birth in the jungle.

They don't know importance of their health. Women have lots of children, 10 or 11 kids. Mom will breastfeed one year, next year get pregnant, and . . . Working in shamba (fields) very hard when pregnant, so become old early. Must have family planning; caring is difficult. They don't follow what I tell them, tell them to come for check up and they don't come. Tell them to go to town for delivery and they don't.

When they see you're pregnant and you are late to deliver, villagers begin to worry. Lots of people come to see their friends if they have prolong delivery. They have fear, death in womb. If I quarrel with her and the baby dies, she blames me, but maybe it was malaria.

Moms eat local medicines, think it will shorten labor, but it's poisonous. Other women put it in her tea, sometimes she knows, sometimes she does not know. I warned a woman a short time ago to not drink the tea, I begged her. She did not listen. The baby died.

When go to shamba during certain stages of rice they need to be there or the birds will eat the rice so women will stay there because otherwise she'll lose the rice, sickness does not matter. Others don't come to the health center because they don't have money. It makes me sad. I don't feel happy because I know health is first, then shamba. We teach them, we tell them, they listen, but the situation forces them to be there.

During birth due to scar get bad tear; this is after female circumcision. They don't like stitches cause hurts, so they don't heal. Shouldn't do female circumcision. They think that sensation will be removed if do it and it will reduce prostitution; women won't want other man.

Husbands don't help. They are suppose to, it's their duty. I tell the women to bring their husband so I can talk to them and prepare them, about rest during and between pregnancies and about money. Husbands have never stayed in the room during a birth, but I like the idea of them staying. I think pains would be less and the husband would say, "This is terrible situation, my wife should only have two or three children." But bigger problem is I think many husbands don't love their wives; they have many wives, so if one is pregnant go to one or two other wives. I don't think polygamy will change. Men with money many girls love because of their money.

Some women come and talk to me. One woman came and was pregnant; I tell her she needs to go to Iringa Town for treatment. It never happened. The woman says, "Unfortunately my child died. I told my husband and he didn't care. They told me I needed to go to town for delivery, my husband says, 'Why?' he does not care. I go alone on bus to town. One lady helped me, but the baby died." Sometimes I don't like their stories because it pains me. I feel like it is me.

They don't use condoms in the village. Women say their husband will laugh; husbands don't like them, so wives don't ask them to wear them. Big number of STI [sexually transmitted infections] and a lot of infertility because of it. Syphilis, we test all pregnant moms for syphilis and HPV. Abortion—it's illegal. Their mothers and elders do abortions. I know who they are. They leave primary school and get pregnant. Parents say, "Why go to school?" It happens a lot and if they have a problem with abortion, they come to the clinic. I do not tell on the girls.

I like to work most with the mother and child at the clinic—pregnant and to age five. Women with sick young kids are given green (high risk) or gray (risk) cards at the health center. Then we can keep track of them. We ask them, why the baby two or three years old and very small, this little weight. Many kids in family and don't have food, husbands don't care; have other wives, always in shamba so hard to care for small kids.

HIV is big numbers here. People do not look sick, but there is big interaction, they are in early stages. One man may run with mother and daughter. Girls are left to grandparents who sleep through the night. The kids sneak out and then you find the girl is pregnant. People do not talk about sex; too embarrassing for parents.

There is a lot of abuse of women and children in this village. Every village is different, this one not much incest, but promiscuity. Everyone sleeps with everyone. One eight-year-old girl left at home with three-year-old sister while mom stayed and worked shamba. Two teenage boys went to her house and raped her for three days. Finally, Mama Flora, one of leaders in the village, heard her screams and stopped the boys. Others heard the screams and did nothing. Mama Flora brought her to the health center; she was torn and bruised. The boys offered to pay her medical bills, that is all, they were not sorry. They will not be punished by the village, this makes me sad.

I have two and three plans for the future—I want to educate my daughter as much as I can, I want my own house, and I want more learning. The third plan of "more learning" is more a dream than a plan; that is why I said I have two and three plans. All depends on my health.

I like to serve, people respect me. People don't ever have a thank-you, it is normal. I know they care.

CONCLUSION

Atu's early life was promising, filled with hope and happiness. An attractive young woman from a strong, loving family, she was well educated and had a solid career. All this was threatened when a tumor began to grow on her face.

Her facial disfigurement cost her the opportunity to marry and threatened her ability to be accepted by others. Somehow, with family support, education, and her own inner strength, she claimed her life back and took control. She added to her family with the birth of her daughter Bertha, and continued to have a meaningful career, and every day makes a difference in the lives of others. And as for her beauty . . . it's unquestionable. Some things remain, no matter what the adversity.

Atu speaks of the problem of malaria in the village where she resides. Malaria is a disease that almost everyone in Tanzania contracts at some point in their lives. According to the Tanzanian Center for Disease Control and Prevention, malaria is the number one reason for visits to health centers and the number one cause of death. Malaria rates are at epidemic proportions; this number is made even more tragic by the fact that it is largely preventable.

Children are at particular risk; in fact one child under five dies every five minutes from malaria in Tanzania. And the problem has the potential to become even more widespread. The highland regions, where malaria was rare, are now beginning to see more cases. It is speculated this is due to global warming; the colder regions are heating up and now becoming breeding grounds for mosquitoes.

The U.S. Initiative to Fight Malaria in Africa is giving new impetus to the struggle. Insecticide-treated mosquito nets are the first line of defense. They are currently being given free in remote areas and at a reduced cost to pregnant women and young children throughout the country. A new, combination treatment of drugs that act quickly are also being introduced as a way to better fight the disease. Tanzania has plans to produce these medications in-country, reducing the price and making them less dependent on other countries.

These strategies are meaningful in fighting malaria, but there are fundamental problems that still persist and must be addressed. They include: (1) propagating culturally salient ways of increasing the use of mosquito nets; (2) providing realistic access to health centers, by taking into consideration travel distances, limitations of medical officials and an inadequate supply of medications; and (3) expanding education on seeking effective medical assistance when ill.

DISCUSSION QUESTIONS

1. Discuss how village life impacts women's lives in Tanzania.
2. How do the variables in Atu's life impact her identity positively and negatively? How does she defend her identity and ensure that it remains positive?
3. Compare and contrast medical care in this developing country, and particularly in a remote village, with the medical care in your country.

4. A lack of education impacts the spread of HIV/AIDS; what other cultural practices and environmental situations lead to its spread and make it difficult to curb?

5. How does your perception of Atu evolve as you read her story? How do you think reading her story, as opposed to sitting with her and listening, staring into her eyes and catching glimpses of her scars, affects the way you relate to Atu's story?

6. Atu said if she quarrels with a pregnant woman and the baby is miscarried, she is often blamed. In Tanzania this might be seen as the result of a curse, whereas in the United States it might be seen as a superstition. Do you or anyone you know have beliefs that resemble this? Do you ever think daily occurrences, or health outcomes, are the result of someone else's will, negative thoughts, or conversations?

7. Atu suggested allowing husbands in the birthing room in order to diminish the pain of the laboring women. Her words suggest a fluidity in the definition and experience of pain. How do you think about the etiology of pain? Do you see it as a biological process that is highly sensitive to your perceptions of the outside world? Or do you see it as more of an immutable reality?

8. The boys who raped the young girl in Atu's village offered to pay the medical bills. This seems like a statement of reconciliation. Yet Atu rejects the possibility that this act was an admittance of guilt, or sorrow. How do you think cultural ideas about gender-based violence in the village, and the frequency of gender-based violence influence Atu's perception of the meaning of this payment? Do you think the payment was an act of reconciliation?

9. Atu said she was sad that she couldn't get married because she it meant she would not receive any gifts. One would think that living in poverty would change a person's relationship to material objects in some way. Do you think this is the case for Atu? If so, how? Do you think about marriage and gifts in the same sentence? Furthermore, do you think Atu is less deserving of gifts because she will not be able to get married? Does your answer influence how you think about the tradition of rewarding marriage with material objects? What if there was a reward system not just for marriage, but for adulthood?

10. After talking about her big dreams of having a marriage and a large family, Atu said the problem of not getting married lies in the lack of gifts she would receive if she were to marry. Do you think this statement is part of a larger, more cohesive idiom of distress?

11. Atu, the sole medical provider in her village, cultivates crops to sell for extra money. In the United States the debate around universal health care

often revolves cites implications on the salaries of medical professionals. How do you think the differences in payment for service could impact the motivations for becoming a medical professional? Do you think this disparity is the result of an impoverished state in Tanzania, or might it reflect a greater difference in perspective on health and healing between cultures in the United States and Tanzania?

12. Atu's mother cried when she saw Atu's face. Atu said she would be a burden to a man who might marry her, and she said children are afraid of her. Yet Atu concluded that no one treats her differently. Do you believe her? If yes, why? If not, how do you think this conclusion might be part of a larger coping mechanism? Does it reveal a measure of resiliency?

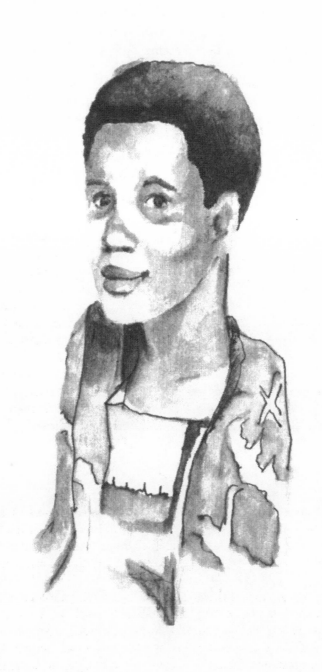

Chapter 2

Yudith

Yudith, like some first-born daughters in Tanzania, bore the sole weight of bringing in money for her family as a young girl. To accomplish the job granted to her by her fate, she found work in the way many young women in the same position do: as a house-girl. House-girls in Tanzania live with families who can afford to pay for their services. Thus, many of these jobs can be found in the big cities. House-girls clean, cook meals for the family, and look after the children while parents attend to other tasks. Because many house-girls are young, they are often seen as a threat and thus discouraged from having interactions with men in the house. Regardless of this taboo, the reality is that house-girls often become involved with men in the houses in which they work. These relationships are known to be driving the HIV/AIDS epidemic, spreading STIs, and increasing rates of teen pregnancy.

YUDITH

I am Yudith. I am 32 years old. Both my parents were farmers of maize. They still live in this village. I don't live with them because their house has no space for me or my son. My siblings are fishermen. I used to make clothes and sell them, but now it is too expensive for me to buy cloth. I sell fish when I can get them.

At one time I was married. The man still lives in the village. He doesn't want to be married to me because, he tells me, "You are too old." What can I say to that? Who knew 32 was *too* old! He now has another wife. My guess is that she's younger than 32. I have two children, a boy and a girl. Betty is 13 and Masuri is 10. This man that I spoke of is the father to Masuri, but not to Betty.

15

I first became pregnant as a teenage girl. I was working in Dar Es Saalam, as a house-girl. My parents wanted me to go and work to make money for the family. I moved when I was 12 years old. My plan was to save money so I could build a house for my parents. In Dar, I washed clothes and cooked for a family. I worked in a house where there lived a man named Ima. He is Betty's father. He was my boyfriend and I loved him very much. For seven years I worked before getting pregnant with Betty. I feel very bad, still today, that I became pregnant. Because of this, I failed to bring in money for my family.

Ima was 33 when I met him. He was unmarried and in school. I really didn't think I would get pregnant. We started to have sex about one month before it happened. One day, I realized that I had stopped getting my period. When I found out for sure that it was true, I vomited and vomited. I could not stop vomiting. I knew I would have to move home to Migori and live with my family. Ima felt sorry, but he couldn't marry me because he was a student so he couldn't pay the bride-price. I thought maybe we would get married after his studies. His parents paid for everything with the pregnancy because my family had nothing to give. I felt so angry with myself that I could no longer work to save money for my family.

When I was back in the village, people would ask, "Why is that girl pregnant?" I tried very hard to hide my belly with extra cloth. But people saw it anyway. They talked behind my back. When they asked me outright, I would tell them that it was not my aim to get pregnant. What else could I have said?

I did not consider having an abortion because I was old enough to have a baby.

Betty's birth was very easy. It took place at home. Only my mama was in the room. I don't know what to say about her birth, it was easy, really. I squatted and dropped the baby into my own hands.

Ima never came to see his daughter. I sent Betty to stay with Ima's family because my parents didn't have any money. We knew I couldn't live with him because he was a student. I was lucky that my parents accepted me. They took care of me very well when I was pregnant.

I met Masuri's father after Betty was born. His name is Haji Mzuku. He knew that I had a daughter but he didn't care because I promised to make a baby for him too. He paid a bride-price for me. This was good for my family.

I got pregnant and gave birth to Masuri. But then Haji decided I was too old, so he found another wife. For a short while, we all lived together. Then he built a new house and he moved there with his second wife. He spent some time with me in my house, but more time with the new wife. I couldn't understand why men here could have many wives but that I had to only have one husband. Why even when he left me alone, I was expected to sit at home and think about only him. So I found a boyfriend, Joseph.

Joseph was my boyfriend for two years. He left our village for Umbaya one day, and no one knew why.

In 2004 I found out that I have HIV. I was suffering very much, so I got tested. I did all of this alone; I suffered silently. I went to the city to get a test by myself. When I found out, I was alone. And now, when I go to the city to get ARVs, I do it alone.

The day I found out I had this sickness I went to my parents' house. After I told them, they held me, and tried to destroy the feelings of sorrow. When I told Haji, he physically abused me. He said he couldn't live with me if I was sick.

I wish I had gotten married to Ima. I think that if we had gotten married, this never would have happened. I wouldn't have HIV.

I don't want to get married now. My health is not well. I am physically weak and I can't do anything around the house. There is no man who would marry me in this condition. Maybe if I find someone who is HIV positive, we could get married.

I am still working for my parents' livelihood. That is my job. This is a hard life, being the one who has to find food for my family. All I do is think about how to keep my parents with food on their table. I rent this little room in this hut so I can live cheaply with Masuri. It would be better if there was room in my parents' house for us to live.

I don't have any regrets because I know that I had to become a house-girl. My family needed food, and it was my job to provide it for them.

CONCLUSION

Yudith spoke openly about the origin of her suffering: the double standard for married men and women when it comes to having multiple partners. Yudith not only became a victim of this system when her husband married other wives, but she was blamed by this very system when, tired of her loneliness, she sought a new partner.

In many ways, the life course of a house-girl is predestined. Seeking only to provide for her family, Yudith left her home for the capital city in order to send money home. When we met Yudith for our interview, we found her in a tiny room that she rents in the mud house of one of her neighbors. Though her words told a story of support from her family after her pregnancy, her narrative left some important questions unanswered. For example, why couldn't Yudith's family provide space in their house for Yudith and her son? Why did Yudith in one sentence say she did not want to get married again, and in the next say maybe she would marry someone who was also HIV positive?

Yudith's story is not dense with details. Instead, it is the many silences, the gaps in her story, that provide us with the most insights into her life and into how her culture shapes her perceptions of her experiences. Unfortunately, the trajectory of her life is shared by too many—it is shared by those who made the only choices they knew how to make, and are now suffering the consequences involved.

DISCUSSION QUESTIONS

1. How have you provided for your parents in the past? How do you imagine you will provide for them in the future? Do you think your culture holds you responsible to provide for your parents in the same way Yudith's culture held her responsible?
2. Ima was living in the capital city of Tanzania, studying to become a doctor. Yudith was from the village, and working as a house-girl. Do you believe Yudith when she said Ima could not marry her because he did not have the money for the bride-price? Do you think there were other factors preventing him from marrying her?
3. How did you feel when you read that Yudith found a boyfriend after being effectively left by her husband? Would you find another partner if you were left by your spouse?
4. Do you think she is to blame for contracting HIV? Do you perceive her choices and her actions as deviant? How does your culture influence your response? If HIV/AIDS was less rampant in Tanzania, would you have answered differently?
5. Do you think Yudith was speaking in metaphor when she quoted her husband saying he wanted to leave her because she was too old? If yes, what do you think are the realities her metaphors represent? If no, how do you think he got away with referring to a 32-year-old woman as too old?
6. Do you think Yudith would have made different choices if she had been allowed to become educated? How do you think her life might have been different?

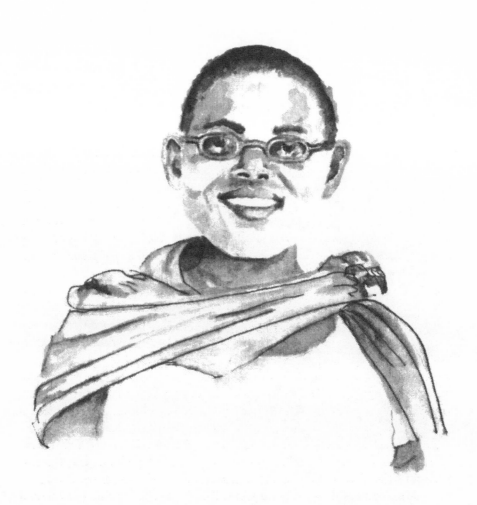

Chapter 3

Paulina

The Maasai are a proud people. In spite of pressures from outside forces they have remained true to their pastoralist way of life. In their colorful shuka (clothing) they can be seen herding cattle, staff in hand, across the plains. Their cattle are considered sacred, a measure of wealth. Their society is patriarchal. Girls are looked at as a commodity to trade in marriage for cattle, and polygamy is the norm. It is not uncommon for a man to know exactly how many cattle he owns — as a pastoralist it is imperative to keep such mental records — while having no idea how many children he has fathered.

In the past, the Maasai had a tradition of killing individuals with a disability. This practice came about primarily because of their migrating lifestyle, which made it difficult to tend both the disabled individual and their cattle. The killings have primarily stopped, but the discrimination continues. Individuals with a disability forgo many of the tribal customs of their age-mates and are usually considered a burden to the village. Discrimination is further encouraged by the belief that the disability is grounded in the supernatural. A child with a disability is believed to be a living symbol of the shameful behavior of a member of the family or revenge by a disgruntled neighbor.

Paulina is out of breath, she enters the cafe at a fast clip, but with a noticeable limp. She is smiling as she greets me. She has a glow, an eagerness to please, and an appreciation of life that seem to emanate from her and touch everyone around. She is a vibrant, joyful woman. We order cake (a treat) and coffee and she begins to tell her story.

PAULINA

My name is Paulina and I am Maasai. That is why I am tall, thin, and dark skinned; all Maasai are tall, thin, and dark skinned. I think my people are beautiful. I was born in the town of Iringa in the highlands of Tanzania and I'm 27 years old. Iringa is a good town, it is not busy like Dar or isolated like villages, it is just right. The rainy season just ended, everyone loves the rain because we know it means water for our crops, it is life. Everywhere it is green and people are happy.

Both of my parents are Maasai. I have four brothers, and three sisters. One brother has died. My brother died when he was one year old. Mama said he was sick, maybe malaria, I don't know. Many people get malaria here and many babies die.

Life for Maasai is lived in the forest in the interior village because we have cows and don't want to be disturbed. Villages are very far away from us, we like to live alone. All the men tend the cattle while women cook and take care of children. Life is work for Maasai; we must always follow cattle, moving from place to place. This is very hard if you are not strong. Maasai men always carry a staff for herding goats and cows. They carry a knife too; they are warriors.

The boma [house] I grew up in was round, made of mud, dung, and sticks, my Mama made it. She told me it took her many days to build the house. In the middle of the room was a fire to cook; it kept us warm at night. Mama, my brothers and sisters, and I all sat around the fire. Sometimes Mama would hold me close. During the rainy season water came through the roof and put out the fire, and we all got wet. We tried to dry during the day, but our clothes were always wet. Everything was wet, it was hard.

Mama took care of our needs; she cooked, did laundry, and cleaned. For meals we drank milk and cow's blood and we ate goat. Maasai love meat. Our best cows were kept in a wall space that circled our house; we had four milk cows that we slept with there every night so the wild animals would not eat them. We protected them.

The time of marriage is ten years old for a girl—I don't like that, it is too young. I'm not proud of that tradition. Tradition of Maasai culture is only for training to marry and to kill a lion. Boys wait long time to get married; they must own many cattle before they can buy a wife. Usually it is old man that marries young girl. When we are nine or ten they give us a beaded bracelet; that is their promise to take care of us. My friend, Flora, she had polio, only a small limp—not as big as mine. No man would bead her, it made her cry. A few girls run away, no one from my village ever did, but I heard of it. They are promised to an old goat, so they run. Their mama sometimes helps them; they don't want that life for their daughter.

To become a woman, someone that can be married, you need circumcision. I was circumcised when I was eight. I was proud; it meant I was a woman. As Maasai we are taught to not be afraid of the cut, to be a fighter. I thought I might not be circumcised because I was crippled, but my Baba decided yes, I would be circumcised. I think this was because I could bear children, I had a value. The village had a big feast that day, many people got drunk on *ulanzi*, bamboo juice. Women held me down while the circumciser cut me. It hurt very bad; I bled, but I did not cry. For many days I was in much pain, I knew this was not a good thing for women. I would not want my daughters to be circumcised.

Some girls are promised for marriage before they are born. A man walks up to a pregnant woman and spreads cow dung on her belly. The deal is sealed. The baby will be his wife if it is a girl. The baby's baba and the husband are eager for her to grow up for marriage.

To prove you are a man, Maasai leave the village at manhood and hunt lion; it shows bravery. My brother killed a lion. He went with other men. He was not afraid, he dressed in feathers, he was very proud warrior. When he returned he told me, "I saw the lion, looked into his eyes, threw my sword and killed him." My brother received a new name, Lempuris, that day. After that many girls were interested in my brother.

Few Maasai go to school. There is no purpose for school. Boys tend cattle so that one day they may own cattle. Girls are for marriage, a father can get a lot of cows for a daughter. It is our value. We measure wealth in cows, the more cows a man owns the more wealth and the more independence. Long time ago there was female circumcision—now just for men. Fine for men, not good for women.

My Mama was Esther—she was middle wife, the second wife, my dad had three wives. Many men in Tanzania have more than one wife, no matter what tribe they belong to. Only very poor Maasai would have just one wife. I know one man, he has 57 wives; each wife has her own boma. He is a very wealthy man. I heard he is building a school just for his children. Those Maasai children will go to school. In my tribe each wife has her own boma, for her and her children. Helps so wives don't fight.

My Mama had very difficult life with three wives, life very difficult for second wife. First wife is mean to my Mama, tells big problems to my father and he blames my Mama. He beats my Mama. She does not have a good life. Sometimes women and children get beat in my country, but Baba beat her often. Now she very old, now no one beats her.

At four years old I got sick with malaria—came to hospital to get an injection, don't know how many injections they gave me. Went to hospitals closer to our boma, in Bagamoyo and Iringa. Mama had to walk a long way with me, no doctor, no nurse close to us. Mama carried me many hours. Mama always walked alone to hospital, no one came with us. There is danger on the paths, snakes, elephants, even lions. No one was there to protect us. They sent me home after a few days, one leg was sick, it was polio. See the pockmark on my arm, face, and arm, it's all from polio. It took my left arm and my right leg. Mama bring me to hospital again—my face was very swollen, got small operation to bring out blood in one cheek. Now there only is the pockmark.

Mama tells me I was in hospital three months, very sick. Mama cried, she was scared and she worried. She gave birth to my younger brother one week before I got sick so Grandma take care of him and Mama can take me to hospital. But then Grandma died. Mama walk and take bicycle, she go back to bury grandma. Mama watched as men dug her grave, they threw handfuls of dirt and put thorny bushes on top of the grave. This is very difficult time for Mama.

Everyone worried about my new baby brother. Grandfather took milk from cows to feed him; Grandfather got milk for my baby brother. Mama very worried. She was alone; Baba was with cattle.

Time in village was difficult for mama and first wife and it didn't get better when I was crippled. Baba go far away and leave me and my sister and Mama. Sometimes Mama leave too, they take care of cattle. When he's home Baba say to me, "Take this, take that," but I can't because I'm crippled. Mama not like how he treats me. He makes me feel bad; I know he does not like me. Baba beat first-born girl, he said don't like her. I was paralyzed child—not beat as much.

My uncle is the only adult in family that helped my Mama, he was her brother. My uncle loved me. I am lucky, in my village everyone thinks it's polio, not a curse that makes me paralyzed. Maasai use to kill disabled because they thought they were cursed. Now that does not happen, maybe in far away places. One boy was left in N'Gorogoro Crater. The villagers hoped the animals would kill him, but someone found him; now he lives with a woman. Some disabled are hidden, they never leave boma. Family ashamed of them; they believe the family is cursed. It does not matter if born with disability or get one later, the family is embarrassed. I was never hidden, but I didn't leave our boma often. I knew to stay.

Mzungu [white people] come to our boma once, they came in big white car. Elders come to greet them. The district officials were with them so we know it safe. They came to see clubfoot girl. She worried they will take her away; she ran as fast as she could, but boys caught her and dragged her back. She cried very hard. Babies cried too, see white face and think it is a ghost. They not take the girl, just looked at her foot and then talked to elders. After awhile she stopped crying, but still was shaking. Her shuka [cloth] was falling off her shoulder, it was worn and dusty. Maasai like to wear beautiful purple and red shuka. Hers was not beautiful. The mzungu wanted to take her picture. They ask a woman, mzungu don't know that women can't speak in front of men. Some of our traditions are not good for women. The elder men say no, they cannot take a photograph unless they pay.

One day Mama says to Baba, "I don't like to leave Paulina here. I want to take her to school." Baba beats me when he finds out I am going to school. I cry, I tell him it's not my idea. I wouldn't want to leave boma, not walk around. I am afraid to go to school; I don't know anyone in school and I want to stay with Mama and my family. I am afraid to tell Mama my thoughts. I cry, but I cry alone. Mama thinks life is very difficult for me, she wants best for me. But I don't think my life is bad. Brothers and sisters are good to me. Other kids talk to me, play with me. We get firewood together.

Mama wanted me to go to school, Baba not like it. My mom put me in school because I had a disability. Difficult for me to watch cattle when can't walk. She took me to school every time. No Baba ever, he never go to school. My Baba no different than others, only mamas visit school. First I went to boarding primary school in Tosamanga. I was ten years old. I am first to go to school in my family. Maybe mama choose ten because time of womanhood and marriage. She thought I not be beaded for marriage.

Primary school is free in Tanzania. Mama take me and leave me. They give me a uniform, skirt, blouse, and sweater. I never have clothes like this. I wore it every day, morning and night. The first night I had trouble sleeping, many things were new. Sleeping on a bed was strange. Running water, bathrooms, and electricity; it was all strange. I cry and sit alone. I say, "Why you leave me, Mama?" I have missionary sisters to live with; they love me. They treat me well. The first meal I got in long line of students, but the missionaries didn't make me wait in line for lunch. They say, "Come around and get meal and sit." I go to head of line and no one minds. There was always food to eat there.

I was the first Maasai in school and the only one. I feel more different. Before I was different because crippled, now different because crippled and Maasai. I worried people be mean because Maasai, many look down on our tribe. But people were kind. People liked me. I can look around here and see things, learn KiSwahili—only knew KiMaa before. Maasai are only tribe in Tanzania to keep tribal language. All other tribes—HeHe, Bena, Chaggas—learn KiSwahili and their tribal language. They learn KiSwahili to unite our country, but Maasai want to keep their identity strong.

Teacher in Standard 1 watches me, he notices I watch, but don't understand. He calls me to him when students leave and then teaches me, he is kind. He says, "I know you want to learn, but you do not know KiSwahili. I will help you learn the language and then you will be able to learn other things." I learn KiSwahili in four months. For four months I cry and I am alone. Then I'm happy and I play. Teacher gave me tea, it nice. Took a ball to play, it fun. This was Standard 1.

Standard 2 teacher took my hand and helped me write. By Standard 3 I was okay. Washed my own clothes alone in Standard 3, I was independent. In Standard 1 and 2 one girl washed for me. No one mean to me at school because I'm Maasai or disabled. I study hard, I like to learn. I finished Standard 7 at the primary boarding school. I am proud, not many girls graduate primary school.

Mama say, that is not enough. Need to go to school for training to make clothes for two years. Mama take me to secondary school for four years in Mtella Secondary School. I was worried, primary school they teach in KiSwahili, but secondary school is in English. I learn KiSwahili quickly, but I'm not sure I can learn English. People at the church paid my secondary school tuition. I learn English. Then my leg very bad, one side comes up—pained.

Secondary school they are good to me, I get to go to front of line, give me small work. There are seven girls in a dorm room. There are other Maasai in secondary school, thirteen all together, eight girls and five boys. In my class there are four girls and one boy. I liked geography and math and English. Whenever I got sick Maasai students give me water. They help me and I help them when they are sick. At school breaks they do not let girls go home; they do this for our own good. They know if we go home our Baba will marry us off for cattle, then no more school.

Malaria, I got malaria. I was very hot, you're trying to study, but you can't think; it's a big problem in Mtella. Teacher gave me a letter to go home to go to hospital. You can't just go home without permission. I was glad to go to hospital, went for one day and then went home to get better. I stayed three months and then went back to school.

I failed Form 4 because by the time I got back to school the exam was over. I was not too sad; I was determined. I came to Iringa Town to work with woman that was working with disabled. I hear about Suzi, mzungu that has a business that hires disabled. I write a letter, bring it to the business, find manager and he read letter. My letter said: "Dear Manager. My name is Paulina. I am disabled. Can I work for you?" He said, "You haven't finished Form 4 so go get letter from Pastor." I did, in three days I was working at Neema Craft. Now I work here and they all love me. Neema Craft hires people with disability. All waiters are deaf; the people that make the clothes, jewelry and art work have a disability. Most are walking problems, many had polio. Once I wanted to go on for more school, but now I like it here.

I work for physical therapy—I'm an assistant. First I worked at the reception counter for two years, I think they put me there because I like to talk with people. Then I went to physical therapy. They like my work. I like to help disabled. I tell the mothers of disabled about my mom, we are an example. In my work I help limbs to stretch and exercise, neck turns. Teach them. I go into the village to help kids. Once went to Maasai Village, I know the language which helps, but it is far and they are unsure.

I tell mothers of disabled children, "Look at me mama. I am disabled, now look at your child." Some say they don't have a child; they hate their child because he is disabled. But I believe they can change, they can get better attitude. I tell them don't close your child in the house; let them out of the house. Give them special wheelchair. Many children come for physical therapy; they feel better after.

I'm not married. I would like to marry Maasai man and have three children someday. To get married a man would come to my parents and say he would like to marry me. My parents ask me if I like him or not. Baba will listen to me, most Babas would not. My Baba has had man ask for me, but the boy had not gone to school. That's what my Baba wants, now he wants school. He says, "You are disabled, my daughter; if I marry you to anyone you will have a very bad life. You need a man who has gone to school." My Baba worries a man will beat me, treat me bad because I am disabled, if he does not have an education.

Now Baba like me; I went to school, I work, make money, make money give my family. Baba never helped me, everything I found and did alone. Now Baba like Mama because she got us educated. He says it's nice. I gave him a cell phone and other things—he likes that.

My leg is better now, still hurts sometimes. I can't walk too far. I take a dahla dahla [van/bus] to work. I live too far to walk. Sometimes when I get on the dahla dahla there are 20 people crammed into the van, it very crowded, no one complains. That is life.

I take care of all my family. Mama lives here now and my young brothers, the 5th, 6th, and 7th born. I want to change Maasai life—I tell them to go to school and they go. I am a good example. I like Iringa. I own land only, but no house. My land is near Tumaini University. Take salary from here, but not enough money to pay for everything. I want three rooms. Now I have two rooms—one for boys and one for me. Pay 10,000 tsh [$10] every month and school fees. I control life of many.

CONCLUSION

Paulina created a productive life for herself against all the odds. Polio, rejection by her father, and the cultural expectations of the Maasai toward her gender and disability made her struggle remarkable.

Besides her optimistic spirit, the three most important forces in her life were the vision of her mother, earning an education, and securing a job. As of 2008, only ten percent of the Maasai population finished primary school, making them eligible to go on to secondary school, and only eleven Maasai females had earned a university degree. In addition, unemployment and job opportunities are particularly dismal for people with a disability. Paulina has proven to be the promising exception to the rule in both arenas.

DISCUSSION QUESTIONS

1. The Maasai Tribe is intriguing. What do you believe makes their lives healthy and sustainable? What negative forces threaten their continued existence? Do you believe that the Maasai Tribe should conform to the main culture in Tanzania or maintain their individuality? Explain your response.
2. What benefits and restrictions do you believe emerge because of gender differences within the Maasai culture for women? For men?
3. It has been said, "The whole is greater than the sum of its parts." How might this be reflected in Paulina's life?
4. What role would extended care centers for individuals with a disability have on the Maasai tribe?
5. It could be argued that aspects of Maasai culture buffer them against the challenges of living in a developing country. Lack of jobs and inadequate housing due to poverty are two major issues that do not affect a pastoralist lifestyle. What aspects of pastoralism would you say may diminish the challenges of living in poverty? Are there aspects of pastoralism that make it more difficult to live in poverty?
6. If your family was living in Tanzania, would you be attracted to a pastoralist life? Why or why not?
7. Paulina said that in Maasai culture a man must own cows before he can marry. Are there similar traditions in your culture? Are cows a cross-cultural metaphor for a common idea?
8. Paulina expressed the idea that as a living breathing example of a person with a disability who has achieved success, she is an image which can bring teachable moments for those who think it is better to hide the disabled. Yet most people with a disability are hidden, leading to the cycling of a feedback loop that is hard to interrupt. How do you think visibility plays a role in education about disability?
9. According to Paulina, in her culture, to be a woman you have to be circumcised. Circumcision thus affects one's marriageability. Does this culturally specific idea of womanhood affect your answer to the questions: Is female empowerment a cross-cultural idea? Can a human rights agenda that focuses on empowering women have universally applicable themes?

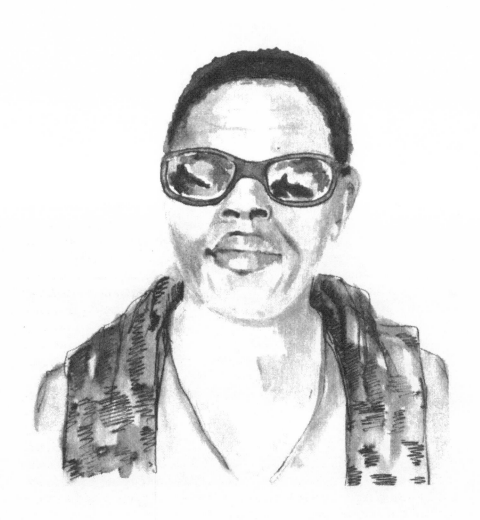

Chapter 4

Modezia

Julius Neyere, Tanzania's first President, once said, "*While other governments are struggling to reach the moon, our government is struggling to reach the villages.*" The statement was made in the 1960s, and the sentiment still holds true today. The villages are the great challenge of this developing country.

Eighty percent of Tanzanians live in villages, isolated and neglected. Poverty is rampant; most families live in mud huts with no running water or electricity. Subsistence farming is the mainstay of life. Schooling is valued, but difficult to attain. Currently villages throughout the country are building their own schools, hoping to provide an education for their children. Building the structure is the first step, but finding teachers and materials must be part of a multi-faceted solution.

Modezia lives in a village. Her poverty is evident; her clothes are well-worn and almost devoid of color. She wears a patch on one eye and dark sunglasses; the area around her eye is noticeably swollen. Weary is the word that best describes her; she appears tired from travel, drained of feelings, exhausted with living. She sits across a desk, arms crossed, leaning forward, her head drooping despite her efforts, almost unaware of the 25-year-old Tanzanian who translates for us. Quietly she begins to talk, her words dragging forward in a monotone, void of emotion.

MODEZIA

Modezia is my name; I was born in Mfinga in a center called Dubulo in a village called Diteta. I'm a Catholic. I belong to the Hehe Tribe; we are a people known for our friendliness. I'm the third born and I'm 40 years old. I have

31

two sisters. Both sisters graduated Standard 7 (primary school), but never went on for training. My sisters are married. One lives in Mwonbuy, border of Iringa and Morogoro; she's 52. The other is 56 and lives in area near Ntella. They both do agriculture and for a long time they have never come home to see anyone. One already has a grandchild.

My mom is too old, she lives in Mdumbaw. She lives with her husband. She still works; sometimes even goes to the farm and does agriculture. My daddy can't work now, he has problems of asthma. He just stays at home. My dad depends on my mom. My mom has hypertension and has been told there is a hole in her heart for almost 20 years now. Five years ago my dad got asthma. He was a carpenter; he couldn't do the hard work. They live in their own house. Not good like a town house, it is a house made of mud.

I went to Standard 7 then studied Domestic Studies in 1985 to make clothes. Priest from a Catholic Church helped me go to domestic training. New priests arrived two years ago. They are new and I live far away, they don't know me, so big problem; now no assistance. After completing studies I didn't have a sewing machine so could not do it. I sewed by hand sometimes, but you need a sewing machine to make clothes. No job.

I was married at 19. My first born was a boy born in 1990, then three more boys and a girl. My youngest was born in 2006. Between my 3rd and 4th born children I had a surgery in my stomach—there was water in my stomach. It was hard on my body; I think it made me weak to have other babies.

My husband divorced me two or three years ago. The problem was the man was having another woman in Arusha going between the border in Kenya. I did not know he had another woman. One day he came with new wife and took all things from me and moved back to Arusha. Husband had taken care of me and the children. He was a good man, but he was a cheater. He wanted temporary woman. We had five children before he left.

My husband left me pregnant with my fifth born. Soon after he left the last baby was born Cesarean. I had no financial resources; I was depending on my husband. I went to social welfare for help. They provided food, medication. No breastmilk for the baby so they gave me milk for the baby. I was so sick I couldn't breastfeed. My mom took care of the baby while I was sick. He never sees the kids, no communication at all. I never want to get married again. I think it's a psychological problem because my first husband abandoned me.

I used to take in orphans and children with disability when I was married. Even after he left I helped them. They come to my house even if I can't help them, feed them; they just want to see me. My husband was not happy about it when we lived together.

Now there is not enough food to eat, we eat two meals a day. It is always the same, ugali [a mixture of cornmeal and water] and pumpkin leaves. My children never complain; they know it will do no good. I cannot work; I sit and I am afraid.

When I got sick I never used a traditional healer. My eye problem caused by two surgeries. I was getting shots, a lot of medication that affected my eyes. I got the problem three years ago. I underwent eye surgery in Mfinga in 2006 September, it never got better and after that I went back to the hospital and they told me I had cancer. All my surgeries in Mfinga till now.

They gave me permission to go to Dar to the cancer institute; they can provide more assistance. I went to Dar March 18 and stayed two weeks. I went to Dar alone, but others contributed money. The hospital was good, because it's private. They give food and gave transport back to Iringa, it's a seven hour bus ride. The main problem is my head and especially right side hurts on top of my head. A hole in my eye so things enter it and it causes more problems.

Those in Dar are specialists, not in Mfinga. Mfinga doctors are so kind, but in Dar so many people that know medicine. Nurses help more in Dar, but they are not so kind. If doctor signs me for free medication because I have no money, I glad. But nurses won't give it, they wanted money. It was suppose to be free I told them, but they do not listen. Medication in Dar—so much better than Mfinga, they have few medicines. Helps me to feel better sometimes.

I had never seen anyone with cancer, but in Dar hospital saw so many with same problems. People stay nine days after surgery and then leave. In Dar they didn't tell me how long recovery would be or anything. They just said you need to raise money, you can't stay in Dar. They not treat me until I get money. I must go home to raise money. They told me to come back to Dar in two weeks. They gave me a letter from social welfare to show people I need care.

I'm here now to prepare money for an operation. I need to find money because it's so expensive. Money decides my life; that is sadness of poverty. Cancer is in both eyes. I can see though one eye, but doctors told me possibility if surgery I can get cured and get better. One eye not highly affected, but with time it increases. Doctors will operate on one eye.

My mom takes care of my kids now. First son went to Form 2 secondary school and then stopped because I couldn't find school fees. He assists taking care of his sisters and younger brothers. Sometimes farms too. Second born is in school—Form 2 government school. Third and fourth born are in primary school and fifth is a baby.

I'm worried about taking care of my children, might lose my life. Kids know about the problem, they think, "How can our mom get better?" My second son is about to sit for national exam for Form 2, but can't provide school fees. I worry. My children not going to school, we lack fees and then without education their life will not be good. It will be like my life.

It was a better life when I lived with Mama and Baba. They were gentle. My parents aren't aware of this problem before. They want me to get better so I can work and get a job. They know there's a problem, but don't understand what it is. They have never heard of cancer. Sisters know about my cancer since the beginning of this year. They came this year, but told me they would not help [this was not said in a resentful way—just factual].

Once I prayed. Sometimes it helps. Better diet helps me. I should drink beer to increase rate of blood in body. But my faith doesn't allow me to drink beer. I drink salty drink. I still live in Mfinga but come to Iringa town to get medication and money for surgery. I go by bus, it takes two hours. I have been looking for money for ten days. People give, but it is small amounts, my need is great.

CONCLUSION

Modezia is exhausted mentally, physically, and spiritually. She seems drained of all energy, showing signs of losing hope. The poverty she suffers affects everything in her life: her health, her children's education, her ability to provide for her family. Village life exacerbates the problem of health care and the living conditions make it difficult to sustain daily life. She continues to search for money for her surgery, but it is a hard battle to win. The combination of poverty, village life, and illness is daunting; sometimes it is hard to find hope.

DISCUSSION QUESTIONS

1. Modezia faces challenges with poverty, village life and health care; which of these do you believe constitutes the biggest obstacle to her well-being? If you were able to evoke reform in one of these areas where would you focus and why?
2. Elementary education is required and free to all Tanzanians, however secondary education is at the financial expense of the family. The monetary charges prevent many students from continuing their education; schooling becomes a privilege of the wealthy. What are the implications for Modezia's children and the country at large?
3. Discuss the ethics and the financial necessity of the decision of the hospital in Dar es Salaam to send Modezia back home to raise money for her

surgery. How does this relate to the current medical and insurance system found in your country?

4. Fifty percent of Tanzanians live in poverty, evidenced by having difficulty providing for their basic needs. What are the effects on health related issues when a country faces this degree of poverty?

5. Modezia said her mother has a hole in her heart and that she has a hole in her eye. How do you understand these "holes"? Do you think this is a reflection of the language the doctors use to describe pathologies? Could "hole" be a metaphor for something else? A reflection of the way Modezia has made meaning of physical challenges?

6. How does word choice in a diagnosis affect the way meaning and understanding are made, and the way life is lived? Is there a difference between being told you have eye cancer or a hole in your eye? Would you prefer one over the other? Why?

7. Polygamy is common in Tanzania. Marriage certificates have a place to indicate the number of wives a man has. Modezia described her former husband as "a cheater." Considering the legality of polygamy, do you think Modezia is making some kind of distinction in speaking of his actions in this way? Would all Tanzania women use the word "cheater"? How does this description differ from the descriptions provided by other women in this book?

8. Modezia said that she never met anyone with cancer until she went to Dar. She also said that her parents have never heard of what cancer is. How do you think these facts impact the support that Modezia is provided? Do you know anyone who has benefited from being the member of a group of people with a shared illness? What do you think are some implications that the lack of prevalence and understanding of cancer have for Modezia's experience with the illness?

9. Modezia said that the sadness of poverty is that "money decides her life." Do you agree with this assessment? Do you know anyone who would agree with this? Is he or she poor? What role do you think the fact that Modezia is living with cancer has on this statement?

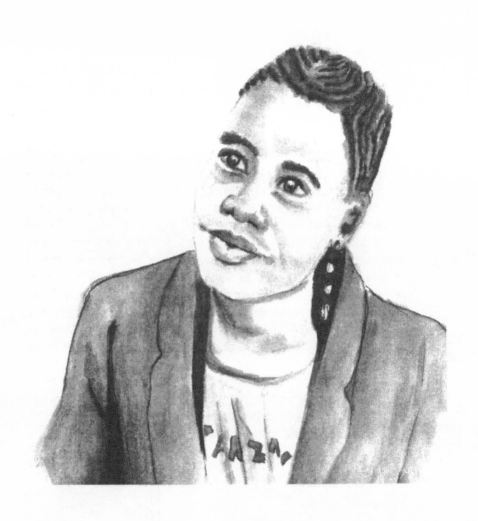

Chapter 5

Rukia

Many people living in the U.S. think of polio as an infectious disease of the past. Because polio vaccines were administered in the U.S. as early as 1955, people born in that generation consider suffering from polio to be an antiquated reality. In Tanzania, however, this is not the case. Though cases of polio are becoming increasingly more rare, a large portion of the young population in Tanzania were infected with polio as children. According to Tanzania's Demographic and Health Survey, nearly twenty percent of children in 2004 did not receive a polio vaccination. The reasons for this range from village level challenges, such as long walks to health centers, to more obviously institutional problems, such as a lack of vaccinations at health centers.

Rukia is the type of woman who talks to you as if you were her sister. Her demeanor is as warm as her sense of self-worth is fierce. The only breaks in her narrative flow came when she stopped to savor large yet neat cubes she cut from the carrot cake we enjoyed together. Her story begins with an experience shared by many disabled children in Tanzania: abandonment. The conclusion of her story thus far, however, demands a sobering meditation on forgiveness. Rukia does more than profess about forgiveness; she lives it with the grace of a feather dancing in the wind. Forgiveness, an unthinkable evocation for many of us, is a moral requirement for Rukia. It is an emotional stance in which she firmly and comfortably resides.

RUKIA

Hi, I am Rukia. Spelled just liked it sounds, R-U-K-I-A. I am 28 years old, and I have two brothers who are younger than me, but I didn't grow up with them. My brothers went with my mama when she left our family. My mama wouldn't let me go with her when she moved away. She told my father, "I like babies, but not if they are disabled."

My father was not able to cook for me. He couldn't go and find things for me either. He was afraid that if he went away for work, I would be alone at home and not well. This is why he sent me to live with his sister.

I grew up in my Auntie Marina's family. After my mama left, my Auntie and Uncle took me in. When I first got to their house, they told me, "Sit there. Anything you want." That was a time before I had these crutches. I had to crawl to get anywhere then. I put little sandals between my knees and the floor and then just slid my knees along the road without lifting them up. That's how I got around.

My Auntie didn't segregate me. They took me as their child. Because of this, I called them Mama and Baba, even though they were not my parents. They still love me, right up till this day.

When I was nine years old I was in Standard 2. There were people who came from a mission in Italy to my school. They were doing occupational therapy. During the time that they were there, I had seven operations over the course of two years. My Auntie paid for everything.

The first five surgeries took place in one day. They only operated from my waist down. Because of these operations, I learned to walk. I had physical therapy lessons with an Italian girl twice a day, every single day, for seven months. She was very good to me.

One of my first memories is when my Auntie took me to school. Other people told her that disabled people cannot go to school. I heard her tell my Uncle, "I will try to bring her to school. All my other children went to school. Why not Rukia?"

So she took me there. Literally. She picked me up, and carried me to school. At that time, I was only crawling, and school was too far away.

Because I started school at a later age, I was the big one in class. I was feeling very shy because there were small children and me in the same classroom. There was one boy who used to laugh at me because I was not like him. Some other kids would look at me and laugh, but after the first year it got better for me. I never once cried at school.

When I was 17, I went to secondary school. My Auntie sent me to a boarding school. I was not able to do work as most of my peers did, like washing my clothes, taking my exercise, or getting to class. Sometimes someone would help me, but sometimes not. I only had two friends who were girls; all the rest were boys. They would carry my bags and hold my stuff when they were around.

At the end of every day, when I got home, I would cry. I felt that I was so far from my Auntie and that I was having too much pain trying to do things for myself. I wrote my Auntie a letter and told her, "*I don't feel that I can live like this, without you.*" When she got the letter she came to the boarding school and moved me home. She was a good woman. A really good woman.

Yes, yes! I am married! I never thought I would marry! When I was a girl my Auntie told me that I would never get married. She said that's just not how my life would go. Even now she tells me that she wonders, "Who, who, who would have married Rukia?" And it's not just my Auntie. Many, many people ask him why he married a disabled.

Let me tell you why this is. Because I am disabled, I can't do anything at home. We depend on a house-girl to do these kinds of things. I know that Daos's parents also wondered why he would want to marry a disabled. They realized, though, that I am intelligent and that I can help out in other ways because I can work with my mind. They want me to help them because they can't do much for themselves.

When Daos asked me to marry him, I said yes, but I told him, "I am afraid to marry you because I am disabled." But he told me that he loved me, and that was that.

Daos wanted to pay a bride-price but my Auntie said she wouldn't take it. She told Daos, "I will not take this because you will be back. You will be back and you will be wanting your money." But Daos insisted on giving her a bride-price, so eventually she just took it. The money is still hidden in a box in her house! She doesn't want to spend it because she thinks Daos will be back for his money.

My Auntie is afraid for me because she thinks I will get beat. He has never beat me before; but I'm afraid, too, that one day he will. When our house-girl finds other work, I am afraid Daos will beat me and tell me to go home. I have a plan in case this happens. I will find a house and proceed to live my life with my child. If this happens, I will never get married again.

When my brothers found out that I got married they were so angry with me! "Why would you do this, Rukia?? You will not be happy!"

"Let me try, ok?" I told them that it was my decision. And you know what? I am willing to take the risk.

And now we have a baby together! Daos and I got married in August. I had the baby in January. Do the math—I got pregnant before we got married! Let me tell how this happened.

I was living at home, because I was in college at the time. I went to the doctor because I had no periods. I was very afraid after he told me because this was not something that we planned to happen!

Daos's sister was the first person that I told. And guess what? She was very happy! She told me that I also should be happy. Because of this, she gave me a lot of confidence. One week later, I told Daos.

When I told Daos, he said, "AHH!" with wide eyes. His eyes could have popped out of his head. "Can I give you money to make an abortion?" he asked me.

I told him no because I was too afraid. We decided I would talk to my principal to see if maybe I could finish school after the baby was born.

I was so nervous to tell the principal, I thought I would kill the baby with my nerves. But when I told him, he said it was no problem! Next I had to tell my boss, and she too was very happy for me. She accepted the situation well.

Because my principal and my boss accepted me, Daos was fine with having the baby.

I had to have a C-section because the muscles in my legs are not very strong. I was in the hospital for one week before I gave birth. When Lilian was born, she was 2.5 kilograms. Now I will try not to have any more children. Maybe I will have to use protection.

My mother died five years ago. Her name was Catherine. My younger brother came to Iringa to tell me that she was sick. I asked him how I could help her and he told me just to buy things for her. But I thought to myself, "How can I help her while she living far away?"

My brother decided to take her back here. She moved in with her sister. During the time she was sick, I saw her a few times a week. Before this happened, I had only seen her two times in my life. When I first saw her, I didn't like to say even anything to her.

She was very kind to me when she was sick. He told me to help her because I was the only one who finished secondary school. She told me, "Help me, my love. I am nothing and you have made yourself something." I told her, "Mom, you left me, you've done that, but nowadays, I forgive you." She asked me, "Please forgive. I am sick. Forgive me before I die." I think she was sincere. When she asked me this, I accepted because I know that God will help me. I knew that when she died, she would go to God.

She couldn't even buy sheets for herself! So I helped her to buy sheets. I didn't ever want to refuse her because I thought to myself, "I can do this. She was my mommy."

If you want me to tell you honestly, I can't say I was very sad that she was dying. I think God knows that my mother left me. And you know what else? There is no place in heaven for my mama because of what she has done to me.

I feel sure that my mama died of AIDS. I know what the symptoms are and I saw all of these when she was dying. In her life, she was living without a husband. She didn't have a permanent husband. She also must have believed that she was dying from AIDS.

I was born with a sickness, not a disability. I had polio and I became very sick at two years old and by the time I was three my legs were totally crippled.

It is very common for people in Tanzania to kill babies at this age if they became disabled. I think they did not kill me because my father loved me too much. But my mama was different. When I was born she told my father, "I can't live with a disabled in my house. I will leave her with you." My father told her that if that was how she felt, she might as well go.

I think she acted like this because I was the first born. My father accepted me well because he loved me like his first baby girl. But my mom—she thought that her first born was healthy—she didn't think I had any problems. So when she saw that I had become disabled, she was not ok with it.

I know this story because my Auntie told me.

I don't think most people discriminate. Because I was sent to boarding school, I learned to talk to many people. If people don't want to talk, then I don't talk either.

It doesn't make me sad anymore that I am crippled. How could I be sad? I have a husband and a baby girl.

CONCLUSION

At the end of our interview with Rukia, we asked her what the happiest part of her life has been. During her interview, she spoke with such astonishing energy for the world and its challenges, that we did not think this would be a hard question for her to answer. Yet this question was the only one for which she had no words. She did not stumble to answer the question, she simply couldn't locate an element of her life that was marked by happiness. The look she offered us instead of words was filled more densely with meaning than a lengthy answer could have been. Rukia did not answer the question because it was not salient for her. She did not respond because to provide a response would be to privilege a single element of her life over another. This was not a choice Rukia was willing to make, and on a very deep level, she seemed confused as to why we would have asked her that.

In many ways, Rukia's story encapsulates what we found as researchers of life histories of women living with chronic illness and disability in Tanzania. Rukia's ability to live in harmony with her reality serves as a profound lesson for all of us. Rukia's forgiveness of her mother reminds us of the value in compassion, and the uselessness of storing our anger for future reference. At the same time, when Rukia stated affirmatively that her mother was not headed towards heaven, she teaches us that to forgive does not necessarily mean we must pull the wool over our eyes— that we can build up our own self-respect by forgiving those who have wronged us.

DISCUSSION QUESTIONS

1. Would you argue that Rukia attended to her mother when she was ill out of a sense of duty for a sick parent, or, because it fulfilled her to provide for someone she perceived to be worse off than herself? Do you think one of these motivations is more laudable than the other?

2. Many readers might feel a tinge of justice to learn that Rukia's mother died prematurely, as the result of a disease, while Rukia, who was abandoned by her mother, made a huge success of her life. Do you think Rukia would agree with making meaning of the situation in this way?

3. Many people in Rukia's life expressed to her their opinion about her marriage that could be perceived as unkind. Would you label Rukia's Aunt's and brothers' responses as unkind? Do you think Rukia found these responses to be offensive?

4. Rukia expressed concern about marrying someone who was not disabled. She admitted that the potential for her to be beat one day by her husband is very much alive. Yet instead of expressing fear over this potential, she spoke of her contingency plan as a matter of fact. What aspects of Rukia's experiences do you think imbued her with this courage? Her culture? Her Aunt? Her intelligence? Her successful career? Her ability to overcome her challenges?

5. Do you think Daos will one day leave Rukia?

6. Do you think Rukia's success in life is solely the result of her Aunt's mentality and choice to educate her?

7. If Rukia was given the chance to speak in front of the Tanzanian government, to influence policy choices that would affect those living with disability, what do you think she would say is the most crucial tool to provide for someone with a disability?

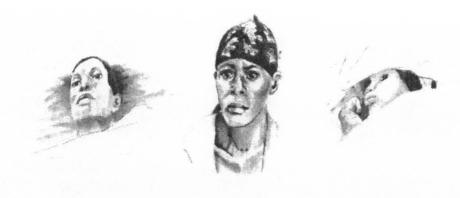

Chapter 6

Dorah, Mbakisha & Latifa

The hospital itself is picturesque; there is a large outdoor campus, beautifully maintained by gardeners. A series of sparkling white buildings, each showcasing numerous windows, are connected by cement pathways. Medical personnel are efficient and go about their work in a friendly and caring manner. Patients' families sit on the lawn outside the hospital, chatting, eating, gaining comfort from each other's presence. In the HIV/AIDS ward there are eight beds to a spacious room; unused mosquito nets hang overhead and nurses scurry between patients.

The stories in the HIV/AIDS ward are all too common. Parents contract HIV/AIDS, their children become orphans and then life circumstances lead them to HIV/AIDS; it is an overwhelming and tragic cycle. This problem is only beginning to peak in Tanzania where some regions have over 50 percent of their young adults infected with HIV/AIDS and 25 percent of their children orphaned. A whole generation of parents is dying, leaving the younger generation to struggle with their future.

DORAH

Dorah is a patient in the HIV/AIDS ward. She barely speaks; she is accompanied by "Older Mama" who does much of the talking. She has thin, sunken eyes that rarely make contact. Her IV laboriously drips into her arm; she is listless as she lies in bed. The doctor translates as we listen to Dorah's story.

Dorah: "My name is Dorah and I was born in 1989 in Iringa Town at Mashinga. There were two in the family. I was the elder daughter and I had a younger brother. Our mother died when we were so young, in childhood. My mom died of malaria. Father had frequent attacks of fever, then he died. They died within one year of each other, first mom, then dad. We were orphans.

"I'm Hehe. I ended with Standard 6, not graduating primary school because of frequent illness. That was in 2002. I stayed in Macambako and sold secondhand clothes from overseas. I did not have interest in this job, but needed money for living.

"Now my main problem is stomach problems. All the time I have abdominal pain and diarrhea. Can't eat ugali, no rice, only porridge and juice will eat."

Older Mama: "If she gets ugali she vomits, bread with tea or porridge are not a problem. Severe diarrhea. Not capable of doing anything; must change her position all the time. Can't sit or walk. Don't know what it is, just suffering from stomach. My life hard too. I live in town; my husband died 15 years past. I have three of my own children. I face big burden. I took Dorah into my home. Younger brother taken by another aunt now. He's in secondary school and starts Form 1."

Dorah: "For almost one year I have had no menstrual flow. Two weeks in hospital now, before this was cared for at home for one month. Doctors recommend I go to out-patient for drugs."

Doctor: "She has HIV/AIDS and needs ARVs. Older mama and girl do not know it's HIV/AIDS. We are still not sure, she is on IV drip till we confirm. She is also taking antifungal drug."

Dorah: "I'm not married. Young and older mama take care of me three days each. My Baba had three wives, my mama was middle wife. Now younger and older mama take care of me. Brother lives with younger mama when not in boarding school. No friends come to see me, cousins come.

"I don't know what I feel; don't know, just pray to God to stop diarrhea so I will become strong. I am happy because I'm under treatment of doctors and in hospital, in a proper place."

MBAKISHA

Two beds down from Dora lies Mbakisha. While weak, she is stronger than Dorah. She speaks in a soft voice, it's difficult to hear, but she is clearly aware of her surroundings. Once again the doctor translates as we talk.

I'm 30. I live in Iringa urban. I was born Nyakyusa and I have four sisters, one died; and three brothers, one died. My sister died, she suffered suddenly and died; my brother had a motor accident. My dad made and sold bread. I went to Standard 7. I'm the only one that went to school; no brothers or sisters went to school. Before I was ill I baked bread like my dad, but illness interrupted that.

My mother was alive, mom died three days ago. She was suffering from TB. Mama had TB—I took care of her; there was severe coughing, sick chronic chest cough since childhood. She died at home. After despair of hospital efforts, we decided to take her back home. All efforts at hospital were exhausted; the relatives and patients got tired of hospital. Before going to hospital we went to traditional healers, hospital was the last thing to try. Traditional healers tried many things to make her better. In village people often go to traditional healer for 7 to 15 years, until maybe neighbor has the same problem. Then they discuss alternatives to traditional healers; then seek help from doctors.

I tried traditional healers before I came to hospital, they helped some. I've been in the hospital for three weeks with a high fever [she uses the word homa which means fever; it is used to refer to every illness by the Hehe—making a diagnosis difficult]. I had an abscess on neck—it started at home, but was taken care of in the hospital. Plenty of people visit me in the hospital—I live with my sister who cares for me in the hospital, but sometimes exchanges with her sister-in-law. No one looks at me with idea of isolating me. They are trying level best to be close.

I was married, but became divorced. I have one daughter, Anita, she's one year and three months. For one year I have not been able to work. I can't breastfeed because of sickness. My twin sister cares for the child.

I can't cope with any foods, only oranges, fluids, and peaches. Pain in abdomen most of the time. I vomit all the time. I feel better than previously. Generally I'm happy, but feel unhappy that I can't eat all I admire.

LATIFA

We next stop at the hospital bed of Latifa, she lies quietly, unable to hear or speak. Answers come from her cousin.

I am Latifa's cousin. My name is Dorambiliny. Latifa is about 40 years old. She was born in the Jombay district and never went to school. Her father is in his 80's. He has no income. He is in the village. He doesn't know about Latifa's condition. We will not tell him because we are afraid he will be confused. He is also sick. He complains of lower limb problems. Her mom died. She had edema of the outer extremities.

In December of 2007 Latifa tested positive for HIV. She has been taking ARVs since March. They are free, but she has to travel to get the medicine.

Latifa was married. Her husband has died; I don't know why he died. He only had one wife. They have three children together. Two finished Standard 7 [primary school] and the youngest is in Form 1 [secondary school]. The children are staying in the village now.

Latifa doesn't know that she is HIV positive. She cannot hear us right now. No one has told her what is going on. As soon as she recovers, they will tell her. Her mental state is changing, so we don't want to tell her now. When her mental state is better we will tell her. There has already been improvement lately. She started to talk yesterday. She is very confused. It was very confused speech.

She started ARVs too late; that is why she isn't doing well. We think she will be an out-patient soon. Her children don't know that she is in the hospital suffering from HIV.

She has one other caretaker, other than me. One of our cousins also is taking care of her. Her sisters were here. They know she has HIV. They are the ones who brought her into the hospital in the first place. The other cousin will take care of her if she's discharged. Then she will live in town with our cousin.

We don't have enough money to be taking care of her, but we are trying. Her cousins and sisters are sad that she is here. They came to the hospital but they were afraid; they are afraid still. I give this problem to God. I trust him to make it go away.

CONCLUSION

In the HIV/AIDS ward each woman struggled to share the most important events of her life. They were quickly tired from the conversation, too exhausted to elaborate. Unexpectedly, as lunchtime approached the mood changed. Families began to appear. Every woman was surrounded by family, three or four members, nourishing them with food and companionship. It brought a certain festivity to the grim setting.

Mbakisha received good news the following day. The doctor was pleased to tell her she was released from the hospital and would become an out-patient, a sign of improved health. Dorah and Latifa, however, would remain, their deaths imminent.

Latifa did not receive ARVs until her AIDS was full-blown and she was very sick. This is partially due to a lack of early diagnosis and partially an issue of when ARVs are administered. CD4 counts (a measure of the immune system's strength) must be much lower in Tanzania to receive treatment than in the United States or Europe. In the U.S. it is recommended that ARVs start with a CD4 count of 350–500. In Tanzania, and most African countries, it is a CD4 count of 200 that is required in order to receive medication. This means the individual has full blown AIDS, putting them at great risk of contracting other diseases. Their prognosis is grim, since people living with AIDS die not from AIDS, but from a resulting weakened immune system's inability to fight off other sicknesses. Additionally, patients must come to the clinic not just once, but three times for CD4 testing before they are given medication. Because of the hardships of cost and distance (to health centers), this restriction is unrealistic in serving patients.

The issue of health care invites a discussion of the serious shortage of doctors and nurses in Tanzania. This scarcity is exacerbated by the fact that medical personnel in government hospitals and clinics are geographically placed at the discretion of the government. Many doctors, nurses, and medical officials find themselves placed far from family, friends, and tribe members, all of whom are important support systems. The result is that many people are reluctant to enter the field or leave the profession prematurely. As is common in many developing countries, there is also the problem of a "brain drain" in Tanzania, because medical students often go to other countries to get their degree and are not enticed to return home.

DISCUSSION QUESTIONS

1. Discuss the cultural practices and economic situations that potentially lead to the spread of HIV/AIDS in Tanzania.
2. Discuss the practice of administering ARVs at an earlier stage of HIV/AIDS in developed countries, while waiting until the individual is much sicker in developing countries.
3. Twice as many women as men have HIV/AIDS. What physical and cultural practices do you believe account for this disparity?
4. Latifa was not told that she was living with HIV. Her children are still unaware. Do you agree or-disagree with the fact that many patients are not told of their condition of HIV/AIDS? Are there benefits to this practice? Are there dangers?
5. The continent of Africa has over fifty percent of the HIV/AIDS cases in the world, and yet only ten percent of the population resides there. What do you believe contributes to this imbalance?
6. Discuss the social stigma of HIV/AIDS in your country and in Tanzania. What social, political and economic factors do you think contribute to or mitigate stigma?
7. Mbakisha went to a traditional healer before a biomedical health practitioner. Speculate on why this choice is made and the health implications. Are there benefits to this choice? Since Tanzanians often seek treatment from traditional healers, how do you think the international public health community could collaborate with traditional healers to prevent the spread of HIV/AIDS?

8. Discuss the role of family in a culture. Does HIV/AIDS threaten the family structure?
9. Discuss the pros and cons of government geographic placement of medical personnel.
10. Dorah said she was "happy to be in the hospital" because it was the proper place to be. Were you surprised by this? What aspects of your culture and experience do you think have an impact on your response? Do you think the ease in going to the hospital in the developed world makes its citizens liable to take its services for granted?

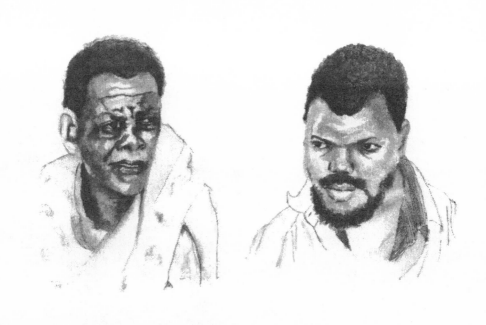

Chapter 7

Madeline & Robert

The psychiatric ward is a relatively small building, approximately 50 feet by 30 feet on the hospital grounds, quarantined to what a Westerner might label the "backyard." The building is divided into two sections: one side for women, the other for men. Each side of the building houses a doctor's office, two bedrooms and a bathroom. A high metal chain link fence surrounds the structure, but oddly the gate is left wide open; people are free to roam in and out. There is a small area of dirt with two trees for walking or resting.

Spit dribbles from Robert's mouth. He is half asleep during the interview. His mother, Madeline, is his caretaker; she sits close to him. Remnants of benches align the small outer patio; they have been broken to pieces by the patients. We sit on the cement as Madeline begins to tell their story with the help of an interpreter.

MADELINE AND ROBERT

Robert was born in a village close to Ilula. He is 25 years old. There were four kids, he was the last born. I had easy pregnancy with all, I gave birth at home. The old ones from village were with me, they are all dead now. I've forgotten the age of my other children [gestures with her hand like this is not important]. The first born was a girl and then three boys. All others went to school close to home. Two graduated primary school, very good, one made it part way through primary school. Dad of family went to Standard 7, like two of his sons he graduated primary school. I never went to school. Now my husband is dead. Robert was five when his Dad died, he never knew of Robert's problems.

I was married, I was the only wife. We are from the Hehe Tribe. We were farmers; our crop was sunflowers for oil. My husband and I worked the fields and when children were older they worked the fields. Everyone helped.

[At this point in our conversation another boy takes off all his clothes, an attendant strikes him with sticks to get him dressed—his body is covered in half-healed sores, his anus is torn and very sore—there is no way of knowing if this was self-inflicted or not. Finally the attendant, still striking the boy, shepherds him into the building. Madeline, seemingly oblivious, continues to talk throughout the beating.]

Robert went to school, he finished Standard 7. Then he started to have trouble after eight months. He started to make this sound, "he he he" breath and hit the wall, banging all the time. He tore his clothes and threw them away. He took off all his clothes like the other boy over there. I saw the attendant hit him. She didn't hurt him, it was okay. She wanted him to put on clothes; it was fine. If it was Robert I would want the same. They need to learn.

Robert lives in a village with me, just the two of us. I'm taking care of him, I'm 35 years old. [As is typical in Tanzania, she doesn't know the year she was born—she looks elderly. Very old, very thin, she cannot be 35.] He can eat and dress alone if I leave the food [wipes the slobber from his mouth]. He can't work, can't go into the field. I wash his clothes. Can't do dishes or clean. Robert cannot take care of himself. No one helps me with Robert.

He sees his brothers and sister. They play with him. They talk to him, not touch him. They give me a little food to help. No kids for Robert, he will never be a Baba. I don't know if villagers like him. He stays in house all the time, sometimes goes out and says hi to others. He does not speak, doesn't hit others.

I have lost all friends because of Robert. No friends or church help. They just left; no words why. I'm by myself. I have no guests, no tea. They came before Robert. I don't know if it's God's will or. . . . We are Roman Catholic.

I did everything to take him to hospital to get treatment. No traditional healers. I didn't know what was wrong. I'm not sure of his age when he started this behavior, but I think around 17 [typical age of schizophrenia onset].

Doctors treated him with pills and injections. They helped a little. He relaxed a bit, but then it came back. Three times went to the hospital. I saw he got bad again so brought him more. He started to say things that weren't right—didn't speak, just said nonsense. Only mental problems for Robert, his body is not sick. He laughs weirdly and cries. He laughs without smiling. I do not like this; it is upsetting.

They haven't told me what's wrong with him [according to the charts he had been diagnosed with schizophrenia]. He's been here seven days. I sleep in the women's part of psychiatry and boys sleep on other side. I sleep with the sick. There are two women sleeping in the ward with me, they are both mentally ill. One woman is violent. We get food from the hospital. The nurses make the food and bring it here, I pay nothing. This is not usual; most patients must have family bring their meals.

Doctor visits every day, he gives Robert medicine. There are four mentally ill people here, the doctor sees each one. The rest of the day we sit and wait. Two nurses always here. Hospital people speak nicely to Robert.

I have no feelings. I am very sad. I've lost a lot of weight. Before I was well, but when this happened, not as strong myself. I lost weight because thinking about him a lot is stressful. Busy thinking about this all the time. Can never turn my mind off worries. Never had check-up, I've never been to a doctor. I care for Robert and my health suffers.

I wonder if Robert will get well. I don't know what will happen to him; I pray to God for him and for me.

CONCLUSION

Some of the most neglected and victimized individuals in society are those with psychiatric problems. A lack of knowledge and resources leave them vulnerable to mistreatment and abandonment. The fact that this hospital has a psychiatric ward is a testament to their progressive thinking. They may be understaffed and under-serving, but they are taking an important first step by including mental health in their provided services.

Robert and Madeline's story depicts the impact that mental illness has, not only on the individual, but also on the caretaker. As in most cultures, the responsibility of caretaker falls to the mother or grandmother. Robert is one of the fortunate ones; he has a loving mother that not only tends to his basic needs, but also secures medical attention for him. As for Madeline, she resonates with mothers everywhere in her sheltering devotion to her son.

DISCUSSION QUESTIONS

1. Do you believe there is a stigma in your country concerning mental illness? If so, how do you see it play out in people's lives?
2. A case could be made that mentally ill individuals are a neglected and discriminated class in most societies. How does society justify the

treatment of mentally ill individuals? How does this differ from the physically ill?

3. What comparisons do you see between the mother/son relationship in this case study and in practice in your own country?
4. List the challenges you see facing Robert and Madeline. What do you see as possible solutions?
5. Describe mental health care in your community. Compare and contrast it with the care Robert receives.
6. Compare and contrast caretakers in your country with Madeline.
7. What in this story is the best indicator that Tanzania is still a developing country?
8. It is very difficult to make decisions about a family member that is mentally ill. Do you believe Madeline is making the correct choices? What elements need to be considered when caring for a relative with a mental illness? How are these considerations confounded by lack of resources at Robert's hospital?
9. How would you define community? Why is it such an important support system in many of the stories in this book? Madeline feels a lack of community—how does this impact her life?
10. In the United States, advertisements for medications to treat mental illness saturate our media. Televisions are becoming more popular in Tanzania. How do you think Tanzanians would respond to seeing one of these advertisements? How do you think overexposure to the notions of mental illness propagated by these advertisements could influence the culture surrounding mental illness in Tanzania?
11. Discuss the multi-leveled significance of Madeline's statement: *Robert will never be a Baba.* Based on what you've read so far about the role of men in Tanzanian culture, what do you think she meant by this comment?
12. How might poverty in Tanzania impact not only the way mental illness is perceived and imagined, but also the willingness of families to care for those with a mental illness?

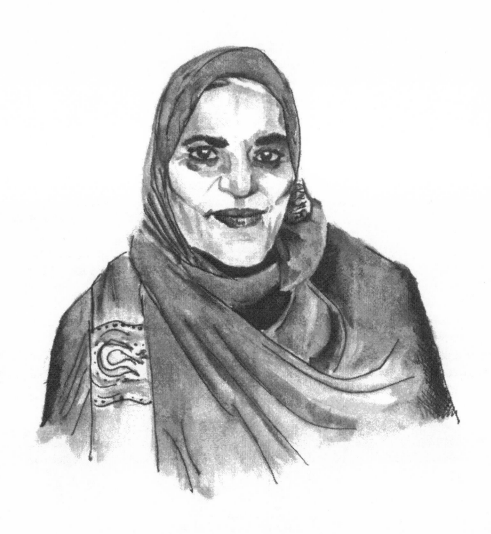

Chapter 8

Fadhima

Diseases such as HIV/AIDS, TB, and malaria tend to make the news in Tanzania. They are not, however, the only diseases that pose health threats. Diabetes is increasing at an alarming rate. The problem is so pervasive that government clinics for diabetics are being erected throughout the country. Currently, at least 29 diabetic clinics, plus 8 in Zanzibar and Pemba, are now receiving patients. Commendably, Tanzania is considered a role model for other developing countries waging the fight against diabetes.

Fadhima lives with diabetes. She is also one of 70,000 Arabs living in Tanzania. Like the majority of Arabs, she has a strong local Tanzanian identity and blends in easily with the culture. She dresses her large frame in a mixture of Tanzanian and Arab attire. Her body is covered in the Arab tradition, but she chooses to wear bright colors with a great deal of jewelry instead of the traditional black. It fits her personality, animated and vibrant.

The first thing that strikes you about Fadhima is her infectious laugh; it comes easily and frequently. She is a charming, middle-aged woman with a friendly, inviting face. We sit comfortably in the health clinic where she has come to check her blood sugar scores, and she begins to talk with the help of a translator.

FADHIMA

I was born in Iringa town in 1951. I am 57 years old. Including me, there are eight children in my family, but four have died over the years. I am the fifth born. My mama's name is Selma, she was a house-mom. My mama is Arabic. She is from Oman. She came here to Tanzania as a girl. Both my parents came here to fight for their lives. They came during the year of colonization.

59

Like me, my mama had diabetes. She didn't go to the doctor as a child, and she developed diabetes in her adulthood. She was scratching her skin a lot, and urinating very frequently. She went for a check-up and found out what this meant. She used tablets once a day. I really don't know if they ever tested her blood sugar. They test mine, but I don't know if they had that kind of test when my mom had diabetes.

She died seven years ago. She told me she felt bad. Then we realized that she had a broken hip. We sent her to Mbege to the hospital there. They did an operation—gave her a fake hip made of iron. But the doctors told us, "This isn't a good procedure. It doesn't mean good things."

After she got home she lived for ten days. She really wasn't breathing well. So we took her back to the hospital in the afternoon. In the evening, she was dead. It was only minutes.

She had a lot of pain, but she never told her children; she held it in to herself. She was just like me; as you see me, you see my mother. She was fat, just like me, but because of the diabetes I have become more slim.

She was a really fun mom. My family didn't speak Arabic at home and we didn't really have any specific traditions. We practiced what everyone else in Tanzania practiced.

Before she had diabetes, she worked really hard cooking and selling spices in hotels. After the diabetes came, she stayed home and the children took care of her. She took the disease as a normal thing. The doctors told her not to eat certain things and she would tell them, "I will eat it!"

My father was Hamed. He was born in Oman. He had three wives, my mother was his first. The second was also an Arab and the third was from Somalia. He worked in the fields here in Tanzania. Did you know that I never went to the fields even once?

My father died in 1970. He also had diabetes. He was so affected by the disease that he didn't want to eat. My mother told him, "You have to eat! You have to eat!!" But he said no.

I really don't remember when my dad got diabetes. At that time it was difficult to have a check-up. He never took medicine; he just stayed at home when he got sick. At home his breathing was very difficult. He got to the point that he fell down, then he couldn't sleep, and then he didn't recognize anyone. It was a diabetic coma.

The doctor came to the house and injected him. He died shortly thereafter.

I went to school until Standard 3. The teacher hit me once and my father said I never had to go again. It wasn't required to go to primary school then.

My mother had eight children. The first born in our family, my sister, died three years ago from breast cancer. She had her breasts removed. She was living in Dubai at the time. She was around 75 years old when she died.

She didn't tell any of us when she found out she had cancer, even after the mastectomy. When the cancer became serious she was in the Intensive Care Unit and my brother called and told us. She died less than a year after her diagnosis. Before she died, she used to visit Tanzania once every ten years.

The second born also died. She was living in Saudi Arabia, and that is where she died. She had cancer, but she didn't know it. She was the first of my siblings to die. It was five years ago. She never went to any school.

Only one of my brothers went to school, the third born. He is still alive, living in Pawega village. He went until Standard 7.

The fourth born brother died two years ago. He was also diabetic. He very suddenly had pain in his arms. After a check-up he bought bread and went home to go to sleep. He said he felt really bad, so I went over to his house to bring him some milk. When I got there, he was dead. He was living in Iringa. He had a business there, making chopsticks.

The sixth born is my sister who died suddenly. I didn't know she had a problem. She just died one day. The cause of her death is unknown. The seventh born is my sister who is alive, living without diabetes. And the eighth born is my brother who is also alive, living in Tanzania. Right now, he is showing the first signs of diabetes. His teeth are starting to fall out.

I am married and I have seven children. I had a first husband, who is now dead. We were living in Songaya; he is from Yemen. We had four children together. From my second marriage, I have three children. None of my children have diabetes but one has sickle cell anemia. We found out in Mbeya. We took her to the hospital there because she was having problems with bruising.

I remember giving birth to my children. Let me tell you, at the time that you are giving birth you don't remember this clothing! [Traditional Arabic Garb] You are not technically allowed to have a man as your doctor, but that is not the law here. I just had to roll with it! You don't think too much during that time about modesty.

Both of my marriages were arranged. My parents were dead, so my uncle found the men, and I said nothing. I didn't even think anything. I just had to take the husband, even if he was disabled! The way we find marriage is not like you [Americans] do.

They paid a bride-price for me, I don't know how much. I got married for the first time in 1970, the year my father died. My first husband owned a business shop. All of the children I had with him went to school until Standard 7.

My first husband was a drunk. He had no love for his children. So I wanted a divorce. It is the rule of Islamic law that divorce is allowed, but the husband must decide to do this. I was so suffocated about his drinking that I went to the head [of the mosque] and we got divorced. Then I went back to my family.

The second marriage was also arranged. This man was really good. He is also from Yemen. He follows our religion very well, and we have no real problems. He loved the children that were not even his. He didn't have a lot of money but he was very loving. He had a small shop for work and I made donuts and sold spices.

I think I was a good mama. I prayed a lot. I prayed much more with the second husband because he was very religious. He made us get up in the middle of the night to pray. Now we pray five times a day!

My children wear Islamic clothes. They identify as Tanzanian, not as Arabic.

We go to the mosque in Ipogoro. All of my children were raised with Islam, but I have to tell you, they don't pray very much. [Smiles]

My identity is definitely as a Tanzanian, not an Arab. I practice Islamic traditions at home; we eat Arabic food and Tanzanian food. Our clothing is the traditional clothing of our religion, and we have songs of Islam in our ceremonies.

There is not a large Islamic community in Mbeya, but there is a large one in Iringa. I have never traveled to an Arabic country, but I passed by some when I was taking my daughter to the hospital in India because of her sickle cell anemia. We had to go to India because they had the right machine there.

In India they put bone marrow in her side and now all is well. She couldn't even walk for one year; she had crutches. But we found a sponsor that sent us to India and now all is good.

I found the sponsor by going to Arab oil companies and asking them to pay. When my daughter couldn't walk, she stayed with me. I didn't have diabetes yet. For my daughter, there was one doctor from the governmental hospital that helped a lot.

The Indian doctors were so great and they worked really quickly. We were only there for three weeks and then my daughter was walking by herself. The medical care in general, though, is very different in Tanzania than it is in India. In India, there is much more equipment. The doctors treated us very well there. We went twice actually, because she needed more bone marrow a second time.

It was two years ago that I found out I had diabetes. I realized the problem at my brother's funeral, actually. I was drinking so much water! My family told me I should check it out, because I was drinking too much water. My brother had a machine at home to check blood sugar, so I checked at his house. The machine said I had it because my blood sugar was a score 16–18.

I went to the doctor and they medicated me right away. I went to a traditional healer, also. They told me to use the bark of a tree. I used it and it worked. It lowered my score to a 10! Just two days ago, with medication, my score was an 11!

I am tired of doing these checks. I have to go to the hospital every two days to find out my score. My brother has this machine at home but I don't have one. I don't want to go there too often because I don't want to interfere with my sister-in-law.

I live now in Ipogoro. It takes some time to get here. I have to get on the dalah dalah [van/bus] which is far from my home.

The diabetes really has changed my life. I used to do business in Zanzibar. I used to take clothes, perfume, and other things to the island to sell at people's houses and shops. But now I can't get any money for my children.

I don't feel that I have any strength. Right now, four of my children live with me, and three are outside of the region. My children's salaries are so low that they can barely help. The children who live with me have their own wives, husbands, and families. So I must wash my own clothes and do my own things. I need a lot of help a lot of the time, but I don't like to ask. When I found out I was diabetic I didn't know what to do—I lost my strength because I know the problems of people who have diabetes.

At first, I had high blood pressure, but I took medicine and now it is at a good level. I don't even have to take the medicine anymore.

Last week I had a problem with my pancreas. They gave me 15 injections. I had pain when I would urinate, that's how I found out there was a problem. I asked the doctor but he said just to take the injections and deal with it. I don't know anything else. He didn't give me any information. I haven't had an appetite since the beginning of this problem.

When I first got diabetes I ate whatever I wanted anyway! But now I recognize that I have to change. For example, now I don't take tea, only milk. Also, before the problem I loved ugali! I would eat it with pumpkin leaves, vegetables, lettuce, chicken. Now I can't eat ugali really.

I started more injections on Tuesday. I feel a little better but there is still pain on this side [she points]. I really fear this side. But now my blood sugar level is 10.

The doctors never actually checked my eyes, but they said their strength was reducing. I can recognize this myself.

The doctors here, in general, have been very good with me, but you do have to follow them around! It's about you, so you have to be forceful. I have never gone to the hospital. Only with my daughter, we went to the governmental hospital.

One of my children is now living in Zanzibar. She was married there. Now she is on vacation in Dubai—her sister-in-law sent her a ticket to go there.

All of my children are married to Arabic people. I would find it strange if one of them married a Tanzanian, but I guess it would be okay if they were in love. But I planned their marriages myself! [Laughing] I planned good husbands. If their marriages are not good, and divorce happens, then it just happens.

CONCLUSION

We concluded our conversation by asking Fadhima if we could meet with her once she received her pancreas test results. She agreed, but disappointingly we were never able to reconnect with her.

Fadhima asserted herself when it came to the health of her daughter, her own health, and her unhappy first marriage. This makes her the exception, not the rule among women in Tanzania. Her good nature, confidence, and ability to contradict the social norms for women have served her well in caring for herself and her family.

Fadhima also faced the challenge of having to frequently travel to the clinic for testing and medication. In rural areas, where paved roads are primarily non-existent and the distances to health centers are great, this is not practical. There are regulations that severely limit the number of pills that a patient may receive at one time to three. Their rationale for this practice is to prevent abuse, but it also results in more time spent traveling to acquire medicine for people living in villages or great distance from health centers.

DISCUSSION QUESTIONS

1. Diabetes is a growing problem in the United States, and it is generally thought that better nutrition and more exercise would curb this trend. Do you believe the same is true in Tanzania? If so, do you think these recommendations are culturally salient? What other factors come into play?
2. Arranged marriages are common in Tanzania. Discuss the perceived benefits and disadvantages of this type of arrangement.
3. In what ways does Fadhima exhibit a positive identity? Do you believe she is a role model for other women in Tanzania? Why or why not?
4. Because diabetes requires frequent testing and daily medication, what are the obstacles faced by Fadhima in keeping her diabetes under control?
5. Compare and contrast suffering from diabetes in Tanzania with suffering from diabetes in your country.
6. Reread and discuss the introduction and the conclusion of this chapter.
7. Discuss the role an under-developed health infrastructure has on individuals with chronic illnesses and disabilities.

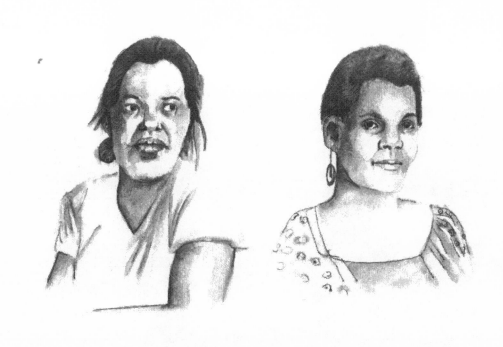

Chapter 9

Luse & Harriot

The family is eager for visitors; they have soda pop ready and tea prepared. The home is in town, owned by the Lutheran Diocese. Electricity, running water, and a television set are present in the house. The father, a pastor, proudly turns on a DVD of a popular religious choir, confident we will enjoy the music. For the duration of the interview, the TV is on in the background.

The initial contact with the family was through the father, Abad. He invited us to their home, telling us his wife had heart problems and that she missed many days of work because of her health. He insisted that his daughter Harriot's health issues were all related to malaria, saying she had been in a fetal position with her fists clenched for years. The Pastor nervously walked between rooms during the interviews, trying to catch glimpses of the conversation. He was clearly uncomfortable.

The family interviews begin with the mother, Luse, followed by the daughter, Harriot. Each voice brings a different perspective to the table.

LUSE

Luse is a small woman, short and squat. She is almost engulfed as she sinks into the large chair in her living room. As she begins to talk, with the help of an interpreter, it is evident that she is tentative and shy, and yet, she is forthcoming and honest. She seems to find comfort telling other women her story.

I'm 52 and I'm from Hehe tribe. My parents had ten children; five of them have died, we remain five. All the boys died, only sisters live. Boys died of malaria and some of them accidents. I was the fourth born.

My mom was lovely, she was nice. She was taking care of us. She was happy with her children. I was cooking with her and she was teaching me how to cook — ugali, tea. [She laughs easily as she remembers; this is a pleasant change from her usual reticent demeanor.] She taught children how to take vegetables, how to wash clothes. She got me ready to be a woman.

Parents worked hard and it was real good. David was my father. Both parents were Lutheran. Dad was a Roman Catholic raised; but when he grew up, he started singing for Lutherans and was happy to join Lutherans. My dad had only one wife. He was a farmer and he has a shop and he was an evangelist. [The Pastor came in to join us, we politely told him that we wanted to speak in private, that this was his wife's turn. He appeared unhappy to leave, but succumbed to the group pressure.]

I graduated primary school at 16. All my sisters did. One brother went on to Form 4; he was the youngest and my parents had more money. I liked school, I liked cooking, and learning language of KiSwahili and history. I liked my teachers. [The Pastor brings us tea, happy to please us; the interview is stopped until he leaves the room.] When I was a young girl I didn't like joking with young boys. It seemed that when I saw my fellow girls joking with the boys, they ended up pregnant. I was afraid. [Laughs] I heard of girls being taken advantage of by teachers. Teachers ask young girls to have sex with them; they promise them money for clothes or food. Girls here are taught not to say no to men and they want money. I think these girls were also themselves bad to do something like that. This is a bad thing that happens at school. It never happened to me.

I liked to sing in choir when I was growing up. I was in a Youth Choir. We practiced three times a week. I liked to sing in choir. Later when my kids were little, and the kids would be in Sunday school, I would sing gospel. Many Tanzanians love to sing, many join choir. We do not spend time reading or watching television like Americans. We like to have conversations or sing.

After I graduated school, I then stayed at home with my parents. I was helping my father with his shop. I lived with my parents until I got married. I met my husband at church. He was coming to the church, greeting me and he was speaking of me. My parents say, "We don't know him, we don't know him." Then my future husband comes to my Baba and says, "I am the one." I was happy. For one year we knew each other and then we married. My mom gave me advice; she said you have to clean your house, you have to cook and you have to wash the clothes of your husband.

I have four children. First born is a boy, he is 30. He is at school at university, he studies law. Second born is a girl, she is married. I gave her advice when she got married — I tell her about take care of her house, cooking, washing clothes, everything. She is done with the university. First born had to stop school for awhile because father had health problems—that is why first and second born at same level of school. Third born is a girl that is 25. She was in Form 3 and had problems of depression so she stopped school; now she's getting better. And fourth born is a 17 year old girl and she is in Form 3 in boarding school.

I have problem of high blood pressure, got problem when pregnant with last baby. I went to a clinic, they have the testing there, and they said it was high. No one else in family has high blood pressure or heart problems. My mom had no problem. [I ask about my prior visit to their home to meet her mother who I was told had heart problems. She denies it was her mother, insisting it was her. Later her husband confirms that it was her mother] I found out when I was seven month along with the baby, they gave me medication and rest. I wasn't afraid of anything, of being sick, I was feeling no pain. The doctors say it just happens when pregnant. They say maybe because of fertilizers are being used a lot, doctors told me that.

I have no problem with baby. After pregnancy blood pressure lowered, but not much. Doctors told me to take medication often. I have to farm and when I do it gets higher. Heart problem, now I go to hospital and they write me medication for one month. Go every month. If gets worse I rest at home. I miss little work, just rest a couple of days. Because I'm taking medication I feel good. If I walk a little bit, it is hard, so my life somehow has changed.

I don't know much about my daughter's depression; doctors say it just happens, sometimes born like this or it may happen when she's 17 or 18. She stopped going to school, during day she was sleeping. We went to hospital in Dar and Moshi. Father and other sister took her the first time to Dar, I had to stay with small children. For Moshi it was me and father. They try to advise her, counsel her. Her hands were clenched. They gave her practice to move them. They say it a problem of nerves. They say maybe she was shocked or something. I tried to find out what was it, but I could never find out. I would sit by her bed and ask her what happened. There was no answer. I don't know, it is very difficult as a mother to not know.

She didn't go to school for seven years. She didn't have any strength, she just slept. She lost weight, wouldn't eat. We tried to comfort her. She liked to talk to different people; today this one, tomorrow this one, then another one. It was among the family . . . sometimes friends. Really until now I don't have answers. Brother and sisters comforted her and stayed near her. Some friends visited when they got a chance. Brother and sisters believed she would get better and be helped. This year she is getting better.

Baba couldn't eat much or go to work for almost two years—he had ulcers, went to different towns for hospitals, he stayed three month. It was like a test, a test for the family. It was better he was in hospital, but he was far away so you didn't know what was happening. I couldn't visit; problem was the transport. [She says a little defensively, afraid of being judged] If you leave here in the morning you get there that night. We have no money. Kids prayed for father and comforted him; they prayed a lot.

I would say, 'God you have to help me'—it helped me real much. I go to services and the program of the week for fellowship. I don't sing in choir now because I work and then I'm tired, but I think someday I will sing in choir again.

HARRIOT

A small, sweet girl enters the room looking much younger than her 25 years. As she curls up in a chair, it is evident she is a bit shy. She begins the conversation with the help of an interpreter.

I'm Harriot, Luse is my mom. I was third born. I was born in Iringa; like most in Iringa, I am Hehe. My mom is 40; Abad is father, he's around 62. Mom is a nurse and father is a pastor. Father has only one wife. I have one brother and one sister. Dad has history of ulcers. It's hard on a family financially when he's sick because he can't work. Mom has heart problems. Brother and sisters have no health problems. I'm most like my mom in the family, I am close to her. I have heart problems like her, but they are different problems.

My brother is at university and older sister is married with a baby. Younger sister is still in secondary school. My dad very unhappy with older sister's marriage, he thinks the boy is bad apple. Dad traditional, he believes he should decide who daughter marries, she not choose. For my brother, Dad said he will advise, he will point to house and tell brother that there is a good wife in that house.

I'm very close to my brother and sisters. I liked to play together when I was little; football [soccer]. I was as good as they were playing. We had a lot of time to play. I worked in the shamba [field], went with my brother and sister—liked it much, to see the plants. Mom went to the shamba sometimes.

Mom was real fun and wanted always to be fun. She didn't have time to play, but liked to joke. Dad liked to joke around too. I like to joke too, but not much. When I have kids I want to joke.

I went to Form 3 in secondary school, never graduated, I was 19. I had problems of the heart—a problem with the valve. It was much pain, trouble breathing too. Had problems for six months before I went to the hospital. I was in pain but didn't know it was heart. Went to Dar hospital, went with my Dad. I was admitted for three weeks. Dad can't sleep with sick person, so he came every morning. He stayed with relatives. Brother and sisters visited. Mom couldn't leave work.

I was seen by doctors and they asked me how I feel and they decide what tests I need. Then give check-up and I need to take medication. I was getting better little by little. I liked my doctors real much. They save me. Aunt cooked while I was in the hospital, Baba can't cook, no man cooks, not even make tea. Baba tried to get a tea list at the Lutheran Diocese, different women take turns. Mzungu [white people] wanted men to make tea, men say no. All women wanted men to wash their cups. Men said no, that is woman's work, my Baba agrees.

Baba got three weeks off work to stay at hospital. Baba and Aunt prayed together. Most scared when told I had heart problem—especially in middle when it was bad. I was really sad to leave my lessons and I was tired of hospital. I wanted to go home.

When I got home I didn't go back to school. Medication made me really tired. No appetite, I lost a lot of weight. I touch a book to read, but my mind was tired. When I'm awake a long time I feel pain. I was home two years. I sleep for two years. The muscles were like stiff in the body from the time I was sleeping. I curl up in my bed. I talked to mom, brother, sister, and uncle. They ask me what is wrong? It was getting worse.

I went to Moshi last year for a check-up with mom and dad—I was there for two weeks. It was a really good hospital. Mom cooked for me. Doctors weren't better than in Iringa, but different. They were really near and comforted me. The two weeks in the hospital I laid still. I did physical therapy. They massaged me, boiled water and put it on my legs and arms; it helped. I moved more.

I took a bus home; it was real bad because I needed to sleep. The bus speed was low, this was good. I was happy to see other regions we were passing. I couldn't sleep. I took tablets for muscles. It got better after six months. I don't remember medical name for tablets they gave me.

Came back from Moshi three years ago. Now it's good, the pain is reduced. The doctors told me not to be frustrated or angry or work hard. When I get frustrated I say sorry and have to be clear to them what is bothering me. My young sister frustrates me; she lost my picture last year. I just forget about it, that's how I handle it now.

I'm not taking pills anymore. I go to the doctor every three weeks. They check on my condition and give me advice. Last time I went I had malaria so they gave me medication for that. I was sick two weeks, stayed home, mama took care of me.

Health problems made me someone that doesn't talk a lot. I think about my life a lot and don't talk much. I have friends and I talk to them. I don't want to get married now, maybe later.

I don't plan to go back to school. My health is not good today. I was up late last night and now I really need to go to sleep. It doesn't go with a season; it's when I do activities; if not enough sleep I get it. If I take it easy it's fine. Whenever I think about my heart, since I believe in God, I have no fear.

I think my life will be real good in ten years. I want to be a success; have a good house, to have a car or maybe cars, to have a business. The happiest part of my life is living with good relationships with people and having good friends.

CONCLUSION

It is unclear what transpired in Harriot's life that impaired her physical and mental health. Perhaps part of the lack of clarity can be explained in the family's practice, influenced by their culture, of only seeing what you want to see. If you don't talk about it, it doesn't exist. As one woman explained, "If you are at a gathering and you see a lion, as long as you say nothing the lion does not exist. As soon as you yell, 'lion' it becomes real and everyone is in danger." This has implications for dealing with unpleasant life experiences. The family has a history of depression; the father was advised to change careers early on because of a difficult time with his nerves. Some of Harriot's health issues may be related.

Further adding to the speculation about Harriot's health are family dynamics and gender issues in Tanzania. In general, Tanzanians have close-knit extended families. Families are a source of emotional support, social gatherings, financial assistance, and caretakers when sick. Sometimes, however, these intimate family relationships become foggy and unclearly defined. This can result in inappropriate behavior, primarily in the form of sexual molestation. Not only is sexual abuse common among extended families, but there is a great deal of sexual abuse outside the family. In particular, teachers have been repeatedly reported to be culprits, taking advantage of female students. The cultural gender bias can leave children and females with very little power or protection over their bodies.

DISCUSSION QUESTIONS

1. Each family member holds different perceptions of Harriot's health issues. Speculate on how they combine to tell the entire story.
2. The cultural belief that if something is unspoken it does not exist provides a double edge sword in health issues and life events; what are the

implications of this philosophy? Have you been influenced by this kind of thinking in your life?

3. What words would you use to describe each of the three individuals, Luse, Harriot, and Abad?

4. How do their family dynamics compare with your own family's dynamics? How do they compare when dealing with health issues?

5. Technology in the form of television and computers are just beginning to become available throughout Tanzania. What impact do you believe technology will have on their culture? What impact will globalization have?

6. How does the strong bond that Harriot has with her family help sustain her?

7. What do you think Luse would like to tell her daughter, Harriot?

8. How would you define family in your country? In Tanzania? How does the composition of the family differ between the two countries and why?

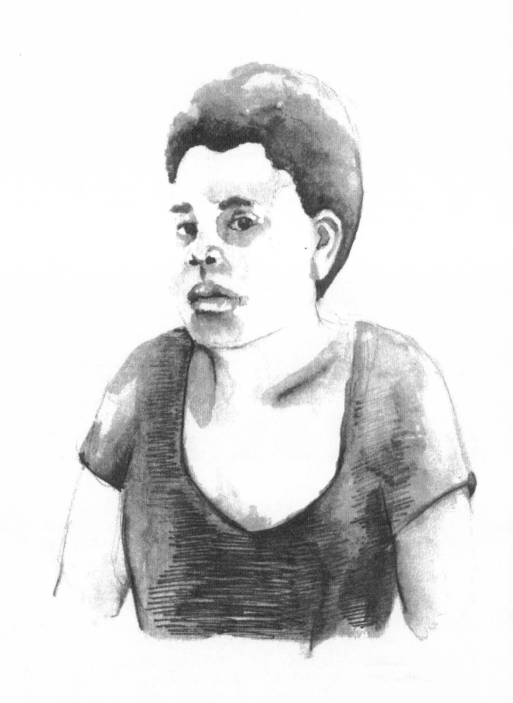

Chapter 10

Maliamu

There is nothing easy about being deaf in Tanzania. Obtaining a functional hearing aid is a reality that is often strived for but seldom achieved. This means that the life of a deaf person is lonely not just in sound, but in social interactions. While there are an estimated number of 25,000 deaf people in Tanzania, the number of deaf children whom the education system can accommodate is limited. Approximately five percent of the people in this community are attended to. Maliamu tells the story of a life that was abruptly inflicted with deafness; a deafness that, unfortunately, could have been prevented.

When we met Maliamu, she had the voice and spirit of a young woman. Her words were sorrowful, but not as a result of dejection. Though there was something sad about Maliamu's presence, it was not because she was depressed, and certainly not the result of anger. Her tone, rather, revealed the influence of Tanzanian culture on the way Maliamu made meaning of her reality. This aspect of her culture can be seen through two proverbs: *Fimbo la mnyonge halina nguvu* (A poor man's cane is not strong enough) and *Dau la mnyonge haliendi joshi* (A poor man's canoe doesn't sail fast). Both of these proverbs express a unique contentment that encourages Tanzanians to accept their reality; they remind their audience that to complain is to waste time, relegating acceptance as the only viable option.

MALIAMU

My name is Maliamu. I am 23 years old. I was born in the village Idosi, near Ruaha National Park. I am the youngest of three children.

When I was very young my parents split up. They practiced different religions, and it couldn't work because of that. My father was Muslim, which means he can marry as many wives as he wants. But my mama didn't like that because she is a Christian, so she left him right after I was born.

When my mother left, I was alone with my father. He was very poor, too poor to have a child. His sister didn't have a husband or any children so she asked him if she could take me to her house to live. My father loved me, but he thought this was a good idea because he thought his sister would be able to provide for me better than he could. I was happy to move in with her because she was a woman.

The problem was that my Aunt was very old and very mean. I don't know why she never got married. She never went to school and I think she was bitter about her life. I was five when I moved in with her, and she took her anger out on me.

My Aunt had a farm. That is how she got her work. One day, we were planting rice. If you plant rice, it is very difficult to handle, so my Aunt didn't like to do it. She said it was too difficult for her. When we came home after planting rice all day, she told me, "Take this bucket and go get some water." I was very tired from a long day so I walked slowly. I had been working all day and I was really very tired. Because I walked slowly, it was dark outside on my way back home, and there were lots of snakes. There was one snake that scared me and I dropped the bucket. The bucket broke. I was just a few minutes from my house, so my Aunt heard what happened. She ran outside, picked up the bucket and started to yell. I don't remember a word she said, other than calling me stupid. She began to hit me over the head with the broken bucket. And then she started to beat me very badly. While she was beating me, the world slowly became quiet. With each hit, I could hear less and less. It took me a while to realize that I had lost my hearing entirely.

I didn't tell her what was happening because I was too afraid. I didn't yell or scream. I knew that I was too young to be yelling at her—if the neighbors heard they would want to know why I was talking like that.

That was the day it happened. The day my Auntie beat me so badly that I became deaf. She hasn't beaten me since that day.

I never went to school. I did start Standard 1 but that was about the time my Aunt started to beat me so I couldn't finish school. The teacher couldn't teach me because I had become deaf within a few days of the first day of school.

My father wanted to know what he could do. He didn't confront his sister because he was too old and weak. He sent me to the hospital. But they did nothing. It was too late.

I also went to the doctor with a different Aunt. The doctor said because he couldn't *see* anything wrong, he couldn't *do* anything. He gave me an injection. But it didn't help.

The day after I lost my hearing, I thought about running away. I knew I couldn't make it though, because I was too young. I decided I would stay with my Aunt, but I decided that I wouldn't speak to her.

When I was old enough I moved out of her house and in with a cousin. Now she won't communicate with me. She says she doesn't like me and doesn't care to talk to me. I think this is because I told people in my new town that I had been beaten by her.

I don't have any regrets. How could I, now I am married and I have a baby?! My husband and I were married two years ago. He is also deaf. Our son is two years old.

When I gave birth to my son, I had a friend there who signed to me what the doctor was saying. I was in a hospital because I live in a big city, Iringa, so people give birth in hospitals. My husband and my mother were both far away, so they couldn't be there. Everything went well, there were no complications.

My husband has a problem with drinking. He had this problem before we got married. Before our wedding, but he was very kind. I didn't think he would ever beat me.

In March last year I left my husband. Now we are separated. I believe we are divorced, but he won't let me tell anyone that he is not my husband.

He had been beating me, maybe five times. He would be drunk and would come home and beat me for no reason. He drinks so often that he has no money to use at home for our family. When I was living with my Aunt, she gave me anything. Since we've been married, my husband hasn't given me anything. It makes me think maybe life was better when I was living with my Aunt.

I have a hearing aid. It doesn't help much. I can hear noise, but not words or voices. The hearing aid, I think, was donated by Americans.

I have learned many lessons in my life. I have learned that deaf people can have a good life. Some have bad lives because their parents don't accept them. But some can have a good life. The real source of life is the deaf person's parents.

I don't like being deaf because I feel that I can't mix with other people. I can't talk to people because when they talk back I can't hear what they said. A lot of people just ignore me, because they know that they cannot have a conversation with me. This doesn't make me feel good.

My son already knows a little sign language and I will teach him more so we can talk to each other.

When I think back to when my Aunt was beating me, I have to say, honestly, that I don't think she was feeling anything. I don't think, even today, that she feels sorry at all. I think she is still angry that I broke her bucket.

CONCLUSION

The most tragic part of Maliamu's story is that her disability could have been prevented. While violence is never acceptable, and certainly not when it comes to children, one can not help but wonder if the outcome of Maliamu's story would have been different if the price of a new bucket was inconsequential to Maliamu's Aunt. Perhaps her Aunt is just an angry woman, and her irrational response was more the result of her nature and less of the circumstances. But one cannot ignore the potential for the end of Maliamu's story to be different.

Rates of gender-based violence and violence against children in Tanzania are hard to acquire; reporting on these kinds of violence is confounded by such a high prevalence—and unfortunately, a subsequent normalization—of violence. Recent population-based studies on violence in Tanzania show a correlation between prevalence of violence among groups of people who are seen by people in their environment as unable to contribute, or as damaged. This places infertile women in the same category with those living with disabilities.

Listening to Maliamu's interview, we could not help but consider how much worse it must be to become deaf after years of hearing. Maliamu, however, does not contemplate how her life could have been different, or how nice it once was when she could hear the world. Instead, she obviates the suffering that could come from mourning this failed potential in a way her culture has conditioned her to do: with a stern acceptance of her own reality and a tangible contentment with her life. It is this acceptance, this contentment, that allows her to live without being bogged down by looking back.

DISCUSSION QUESTIONS

1. Have you ever allowed overwhelming stress to mediate how you treat others?
2. Do you know anyone whose capacity to parent is hindered by grave circumstances such as living paycheck to paycheck, or the loss of a job? Does this story change how you might relate to someone in a different socioeconomic class than yourself?

3. There are many actors in this story who could have potentially changed the outcome: Maliamu's Aunt, her father, the doctor, the school teacher. How do you think they could have acted differently if they had access to a different set of tools or skills?

4. Based on your response to question 3, how do you think international public health organizations could best prevent a situation like this from re-occurring?

5. Do you think Maliamu's husband would have failed to take seriously the responsibility of providing for his wife if she was not deaf?

6. The two reasons Maliamu reported that prevented her from speaking up when her Aunt was beating her were (1) the hierarchical relationship between Maliamu and her Aunt because of their age; and (2) her perception that her neighbors would judge her for yelling at her Aunt. If this situation was occurring in the United States, do you think a child would be influenced by the same factors? If not, what factors do you think would influence their response?

7. The deaf community in the United States is large and unified. Their collective argument fights against the rising popularity in cochlear implants by rejecting the notion that the way they experience the world is abnormal. Instead, they assert that their lived reality should be embraced, rather than altered. Do you think Maliamu would agree with this argument? If not, what are the material differences in the culture of the deaf community in the United States and Maliamu's culture that would prevent her form aligning herself with them?

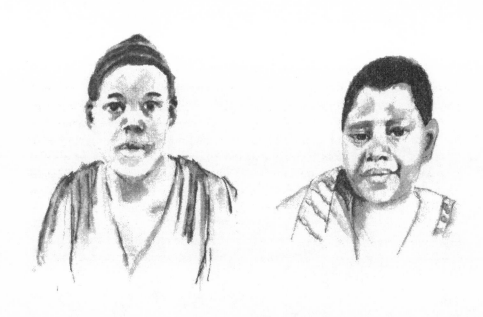

Chapter 11

Maua & Isabella

Tanzania ranks number fourteen among countries in the world with the highest incidence of tuberculosis (TB). TB is an infectious disease that usually attacks the lungs causing chest pain and cough, although it may travel throughout the body. Wherever it resides, it is a potential killer. The incidence of HIV/AIDS contributes significantly to the transmission of TB. In a country such as Tanzania, where HIV/AIDS rates are high, the two unite to make a deadly combination. Though TB is highly treatable, its marked prevalence in the developing world reveals how illnesses that affect the wealthy are often a higher priority for global health action than those affecting the poor.

The lightly smoke-filled room is crowded with chronically ill women. There are at least 20 women in the house, the majority of whom are desperately poor and have TB. It is a shocking scene. They sit covered by their kanga, waiting to share their story, wanting to be heard.

MAUA

In a corner sits Maua, she is a timid little creature; a pretty young woman, but every movement she makes is painful. She is 28 years old, but her body resembles that of an old woman. She can barely walk and needs the assistance of a friend. She has a conga draped over her, but even so you can tell she is extremely thin. With the aid of an interpreter, Maua begins to speak.

I was born in Iringa—I had one brother who went to Standard 4 and one sister who went to Standard 7, but they are younger than me. I'm Christian and HeHe. Rosa Abumo was my mom, she died, but I don't know why. I was very little. When I was little I was happy because I had one parent alive.

81

Baba was a driver. He had four wives, my mom was first wife. No other wife helped once Mom died. Baba also died—I heard it was from fever, but don't know for sure. After Baba died I had a bad life.

Grandmother took care of us. She was sometimes good, sometimes bad. She gave us nice food, helped us for a certain time and then refused to help. She was tired, Grandmother had all three of us and my uncle's kids to take care of—there were five altogether.

I went to Standard 7 primary school while with Grandmother. I graduated at 15. I left the home when I was 15 and went to be a house-girl. I did not want to go, but Grandmother did not want me to stay. I was house-girl for Mmas in Iringa. I didn't like it, wanted to be with young brother and sister. Truly he was helping me. I'd wake up in the morning, wash floors, wash dishes, cook all the meals, wash clothes. I worked hard, very hard life. House-girls not respected, people beat you and use you. Men force girls to sleep with them or give 1,000tsh [$1]; girls agree, they need money to buy clothes, to eat.

This is the fourth year of being sick. It started with one finger in pain, then whole hand, then legs. I get fatigue. I went to the hospital. Doctors told me I had joint problem. I got medicine, it helped a little, but the problem is still there.

Now I go to doctors often. I have TB of the bones. I don't know how it works, they haven't told me. They give me medication. [It is common for doctors and other medical officers to explain very little to patients; diagnosis and treatment are accepted in blind faith by the patient.] I go once per week. First told I would get medicine and physical exercise, but I've never received physical exercise. My fingers won't open, I walk in pain with legs and they won't go straight. When I found out I had TB I felt fear, but I had hope there was a way to get rid of the problem.

I'm not married. I have one child, a girl, Annette. She is 11 years old; I was 17 years old when I gave birth. I was working as house-girl. I have no marriage plans; all men will be the same—give you a baby and then run away like the first one did. The father is not there. Annette is still schooling so she can't help me. She stays with others. I am sad that she does not live with me. Annette is small and just feels bad that I am sick. She doesn't worry about helping her mom in the future yet, she's too young.

I have no work. I can do nothing because my arm and leg won't move. I will work if I heal, but I don't have a special type of work or skill.

My aunt helps me, I live with her. She gives me food, the medicine is free. I'm feeling better except one leg is in constant pain. I still have friends and they are good to me. The doctors and nurses are also good to me. Life is hard, but I am thankful people are good to me.

ISABELLA

Isabella is desperate for money; repeatedly she makes a case for needing money to buy milk to improve her health. She is of average height and weight, but there is a drawn look on her face; her hands are continually tense, expressing her desperation.

My name is Isabella. I was born in Mkete District and I'm 45 years old. My mother died in 1970. I was a juvenile, just growing. My mother had nine children; I was the first born. When having labor of last child mama died, but last born lived. She was in hospital in Mkete delivering the baby when she died. She was a farmer and the family also helped with cultivation. When I was young I liked working on the farm.

Dad died in 1988. He was a driver. He had a headache, went to the hospital and the same day died—no one knows why. Dad was very good, took care of all of us after mom died. He only had the one wife. He made sure I went to Standard 7 and then I was married; now I have four children.

I have three girls and one boy. All were born in the hospital in Iringa Town. Easy births, nurses were with me. My husband sent me to the hospital with a car [proud of this, it showed his money and love]. They all stayed with me, my children. Two are married and one finished Standard 7, but didn't continue because of financial conditions, and one is a dahla dahla [small bus] conductor.

My husband died in 1999—blood coming from his nose and then he died. My husband was a driver like my dad. I don't want to marry again—it's enough to take care of my children, it's enough for me. I'm from the Kinga tribe, my husband was Bena. All my children are Bena, children take tribe from Dad. In Kinga tribe when husband dies, the wife doesn't remarry. Most in Mkete district are Kinga. Mkete district is traditional, everyone is circumcised; it is a secret that is true. No condoms sold in Mkete. We are hard workers. We have many orphans, many parents die.

There were two wives, and I was the second. At first my husband hid he had a first wife, but when first wife separated from him she brought their kids to me. I surprised, but took kids in and cared for them. After he died the first wife came to stay with me. It was my idea to have her move in with her two children. She never told me why she and our husband separated. We took care of the kids together and still live in the same house. We love each other.

At first I didn't know what I had when I got sick. Then I found out I had TB of the lungs. The problem started in 2000, I was brushing my teeth; a lot of blood was coming out. Doctors measured and said I had TB and I started getting treatments. I was surprised when I was told I had TB. They said I must have milk everyday; hard economic situation to buy milk with no husband.

When I don't get milk for two days the blood comes when I brush my teeth and my chest feels like fire. I was told to take medication two times a day and drink milk. I stay at home.

I was told not to work, so I'm poor; it is difficult to buy milk. I have been told everything by doctors and nurses that is needed. Doctors and nurses are good to me. I never want to ask doctors why I have TB. I like to ask doctors why am I taking this medication and not getting better. One day I said to a doctor maybe I have HIV. Doctor says to go check. I did, but I only have TB. I wasn't scared to take HIV test because I wanted to know the problem. I believe if I have milk and medication I can be cured, I'll get better [she appeared to have HIV/AIDS].

First wife works more because of my illness. She sends me to the hospital when I need to go. I still have friends, they don't leave me. My children are not scared of me. No one told me it might be contagious.

When I was not sick I was happy. Now I feel bad because of the pain. Cold weather makes it worse. Only chest pain. I can walk to the market. Smoke when cooking pains me, I cook over charcoal in my kitchen; smoke fills my lungs.

Toughest time in life is now when I'm sick. I would like to have studied and then worked, but got married early at 20. My daughters married early, one married at 20 and one at 22. I was happy for them because I had no ability to send them to school, so could serve the two boys if I didn't have to worry about the girls. If they had been able to go to school it wouldn't have been good to get married early. I am a good mom.

CONCLUSION

Maua, like so many female orphans in Tanzania, became a house-girl. Boys who are orphaned often end up as street children, a fate desired over that of the house-girl. Once girls are orphaned, they can be claimed by families to work as virtual servants. The house-girls' low status and high physical and sexual abuse rates make it a profession with a great deal of potential risk.

The TB that these women suffer from adds to the complexity of their lives. Tanzania has a strong cultural tradition of family taking care of family. Maua is lucky to benefit from that tradition; her aunt is helping care for her. Isabella found a creative way to handle her situation by inviting the first wife to move in with her. While a first wife could be considered family, many women would not view this as a desirable option; however, for these two women it worked.

Unfortunately, the health issues that now face Tanzania are putting an unbearable strain on families. Caring for extended family is becoming too heavy a burden for the living and the healthy. Grandmothers, in particular, are raising three, four, and even five families' children under one roof. They are exhausted and overwhelmed; often not able to supply the basic needs of food and clothing or the structure that children benefit from. The next generation is paying a high price for not having their parents' guidance.

DISCUSSION QUESTIONS

1. What did you find most interesting about these stories?
2. Walking into a home, literally filled with women that were ill, was one of the most emotional events of gathering information for this book. Why do you believe so many women wanted to tell their story?
3. It could be said that grandmothers are holding the country of Tanzania together, but they are becoming overworked and overwhelmed. What do you believe can be done to lighten their load? Do you see this trend in any other cultures?
4. Discuss the plight of house-girls. What aspects of Tanzanian culture do you believe contribute to the gender differences in this developing country?
5. As these women suffer, life goes on for all those around them, how does this juxtaposition impact those with illness?
6. Discuss the positive and negative role of community in the lives of women with chronic illnesses and disabilities.
7. What did you learn about yourself from reading this chapter?
8. Isabella said, "I don't want to marry again—it's enough to take care of my children, it's enough for me." What does this statement reveal about the role of marriage in a Tanzanian woman's life? Could you imagine a divorced friend of yours saying something like that?
9. What was your first reaction when you read that Isabella took care of children of her husband's first wife? Did you have a similar response when you read that the co-wives moved in together after their husband died? What aspects of the way marriage functions in your culture are revealed by your response?

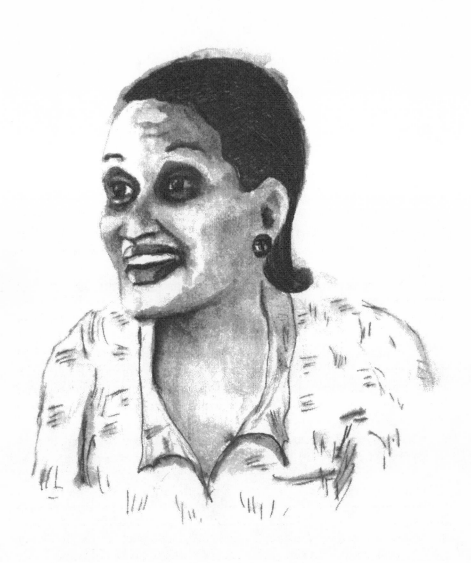

Chapter 12

Faustina

Individuals with spinal cord injuries are some of the most marginalized in the country of Tanzania. The main cause of spinal cord injuries is vehicular accidents, although falling from heights while picking fruit, tripping while carrying baskets on one's head, and TB of the spine also account for a number of the injuries.

Research is limited, but it appears that approximately 1,380 spinal cord injuries occur each year in Tanzania. Only 100–120 of those receive any hospital treatment. Of those lucky enough to have access to a hospital, additional complications often take their lives. The problems continue to mount for those who survive. Since the country is struggling to make sure its citizens are fed, one could predict that rehabilitation centers are rare, wheelchairs are expensive, and roads are inaccessible. With all of these factors combined, individuals are considered fortunate to live two years after this type of injury.

FAUSTINA

Faustina sits comfortably in a wheelchair behind her desk at work. She laughs frequently and is a world-class storyteller, articulate and charming. She is joyful and engaging, charisma spills from her. During her story people enter and leave the room. Faustina greets each one, making all feel welcome. Her story took almost no prompting; she laughed, she cried, she embraced her life as she talked at a fast clip.

I remember growing up. I had a loving family, many good memories. We are all girls, not good to have only girls. People would think we would

87

become prostitutes, because we would need money. One day my uncle came to our house and wanted us to become circumcised. My father chased him from the house and said no one will do this to my daughters. He was proud to have daughters. Mama had to work very hard because dad was gone much of the time. Dad was in Mtinga. He was a business man, he had a very big shop selling cloth. He was a tailor also; he was teaching people how to tailor. He came home a few times a year, this is not unusual. We lived in a village close to Moshi. It was nice, a good place.

During Christmas time my mama was very busy. My dad came home at Christmas time. Mama would write to him, "Do not forget to bring dresses home for your daughters for Christmas." I can remember sitting together and Mama opened box with the gifts and started giving dresses, she would say, *this one is for you, this is yours, daughter this is yours. Put it on, let me see. Do you like it?* I remember during Christmas Baba use to kill chicken for dinner, he called my Uncle to get chicken. My mama I remember how busy she was cooking. One week before Christmas she cleaned house.

My mama and sisters, we cooked together. Mama would say, "Make sure you are very clean when you are cooking. Make sure and when you are eating do not eat with your mouth open." I remember it very much, her saying, "Suzi, close your mouth. So that when we are together we can look at Suzi." She used to tell us we have to eat breakfast. I remember after this moment we take our dinner at 7:00 or 7:30. I was talking with my sisters, she say, "remember how mama told us so don't forget to be clean and how to cook. Faustina you are a mother so remember to tell your daughter." I remember.

One Easter—I can't forget—my father bought shoes for my mother, just the color of your shirt, very bright blue. I am little, but by now I know how to write mama and baba. My mama was in preparing herself, she has on her dress ready to go to church, but while she was preparing herself I wrote "mama" on her shoes. When she came out she was upset when she saw the shoes, she said, "Baby, how can you do this to me?" I say, "I'm sorry," she say, "Don't say sorry to me, now I am late for church." My mommy so kind, other children run from home to get my uncle. My older brother [uncle], he says, "No mama, don't be upset mama, I know what to do. I come with kerosene and clean the shoes." [Laughs]

And then I remember when I was seven also I had encephalitis. I couldn't walk or do anything. So my mama would carry me [she begins to weep in gratitude for her mother's kindness]. Do you know what? When she passed away I thought, oh my God please, please let her be here again. I remember how she carried me all the time, she was so sweet. That time when I was sick I can't get sleepy, I am pain all the time, I cry all the time. My legs were not working. I had therapy and then at that time she was always there. I was in the hospital; I was there for six months [this is said matter-of-factly and is not considered a lengthy stay]. I was with my sister at the end, my mama gave birth to her last child. That baby, she was beautiful that girl, I can tell you. She is a beautiful girl, you know, just like my mama.

I have very much pain, I went home from hospital but was suffering in the spine. My dad came back to our village; he decided to send me to another hospital. There I had a very big operation, it helped, but you know what, after that I still feel pain, pain, pain. I don't know what happened, my family worried. Mama do everything so I can survive, teach me how to fight. You do not have to die, she tells me. They operate on me seven times. I say, No mommy, now I die. She say, No you will not die, you will live until you have your own child [she smiles at the tender memory].

My mama wants me to be saved; I remember I get confirmation in Lutheran. In Roman Catholic called communion, but I'm Lutheran. I remember one thing, in town I got a chance to make a choice, because my mama thought I would die. So I remember when I was going home from church, I think, Oh thank you God, now if I die I will be saved. When I am on the way from the confirmation, I say oh thank you God, now if I die I am happy because Faustina is a big girl. At this time I am grown up.

Very much, my family values school. My mother's generation went to 8th grade [laughs] and so did my dad, 8th grade also. I can remember my mother's handwriting—it was nice, it was like using a computer, it was wonderful. Have you tried writing like a computer? It was nice; I can see it in my mind.

Well, you know; I remember I finished Form 4 in boarding school in Tanga and finished in 1992. Since that time I was going to school and then back to home; went to Mbeya, to Dar es Salaam and then back to Moshi. When I finished Form 4 I was selected to go to Mbeya to study agriculture, but you know what? I didn't make it, I didn't make it. [laughs in surprise] I told my Baba, I can learn something else, but I do not like agriculture. I said, I can't stay here, it's very cold, can't stay here. My father listened to me so much. Most fathers would not. My father says, "What you want?" I say, "I want to be a secretary," so I go to Dar to learn secretarial and computer. I stay with my aunt there. I went to computer school for one year and learned Microsoft and Excel. Yes, it is true, I can use computer. [pride] During that time I would go to offices to work, then to Moshi to visit my father and Tanga to visit my sister. Tanga is beautiful. I didn't like Dar as much as Tanga—traffic is terrible, people shout, it is crazy.

My father loves us so much. When my mama passed away, we think he needs another woman, but he himself thinks, no, I have my children. We children talk together, then go to him and say, You cannot live like this, you need a wife. He says, I will not get married. So we say, Baba, you need wife.

He laugh, he say, "No, no, no, I don't want to marry a woman, then when you come home during the Christmas or holiday they will say no they do not want you in my home, do this or don't do that. I love you and want you to come home and be happy." He cared about us so much.

My dad died of cancer, it was bladder. He suffered long, two years. My sister Mary is the one who took care of him and then he died. She is working on the farm at the home. Mary is very strong woman, very, very strong. Mary, she is second born; even my mother and father when they say, "You know what Mary, you look like you are strong like a man."

Then I come to Moshi in 2002, so I went and I got the job and do you know what, it didn't last, because then I got the spinal cord injury. [laughs] I was in the accident and I could not do it. I was in Mwanga on our way to Moshi from Dutes; we were passing a car and there was an accident. It was a terrible accident I was sitting in the front and I went through the window in the car. Others come to carry me. I can't feel my legs, I thought my God this is the end of my time. I have never had a gun in my life, but I was looking around, feeling my body frantically, searching for the gun to shoot myself. But when I can't feel my legs and I say no, I must die now! I was outside the car awake.

I remember how they carry me to transport me to the car to get me to another town. They call my family to tell them. I remember everything. Others had minor injury. They look after their injuries quickly. They put me in a truck, they picked me up; but you know what, because God was with me, they took me and lie me on the seat and transport me very carefully to hospital and they call the YMCA. It was with God's help they took me to the hospital. I see the doctor and tell him I can't feel my legs, I can't feel my legs! He says, You have a spinal cord injury. I know nothing about a spinal cord injury. I know nothing about spinal cord injury. I remember how doctors and nurses come to see me, they say, "Ohhhhh pole [sorry], she is beautiful, she is too young." But I don't get the picture of why they feel sorry.

I don't understand why this is happening, I do not know what is going on. I think after three months I will stand up and walk. My father comes to visit me, and he cries. I suppose he cries all the time; my father was told his daughter will not walk. He is not happy anymore. Later my sisters told me the family cry. Then they told me, my father use to call me by my childhood name, Habina. "Oh Habina has been suffering hard my daughters. I remember how she suffer with encephalitis and now she suffer with this." Sometimes I feel like while my dad died of cancer, he died because he sad about me.

So I was staying in bed and God gave me very good sisters, they are my hope, they look after me. I never got bed sores! [this is said in amazement and with pride] And you know what? After a month my breasts got very big and my sister go to the doctor and ask why? Doctors said this happens when a person suffers spinal. They tell them I am vomiting and menstruation is stopped like I am pregnant, but they say, "she is not pregnant, do not be afraid."

Then doctors take me for ultrasound and they say, "Oh Faustina, there is a child." I began big shouting—aaaaaah. [laughs] I feel crazy. My older sister opens the door, and says what is going on in here. Because I can't stand up I end up on the bed shouting. So what am I going to do now? Doctors say, "Praise the lord, you have a child." I say, "No, I do not want one." Even my sister encourages me to not have child, because doctors already tell her that I will never stand up again. I still do not understand.

The way I found I would not walk still angers me. A doctor from another country says, "You know what?" I say, "No." He says, "You have spinal cord injury and you will never stand up again." He blurts it out, not caring. I scream "get out of my room I never want to see you again." I hate him. Then I didn't believe him, I denied. So I say no, I will have abortion, I do not want this child, I will not be able to care for her, what will she think of her mama. No. At the same time, I do not think I am disabled, I will not admit.

I call my sister and tell her I do not want a baby. She say, "I will do whatever you want Faustina, that I will do." So my sister goes to get a doctor, it was the one that took care of my leg when I was a child. He does not recognize me, but I recognize him. He did surgery on my leg. I tell doctor, "I am pregnant," he says, "Praise the lord," my sister says, "What?" He says, "this is good news, sit down and I will tell you why, because of this Faustina will have reason to live." My sister tries to tell him my situation. He tells her more about spinal cord injury and says, "Please don't try to abort the child, this is the reason she will live." My sister comes to me and tells me doctor refused, I say, "this doctor hates me, he hates me, he wants me to be an experiment." My sister says, "No, no."

I go to other doctors, they all say, "No, we do not kill." I was crazy talking to every doctor, but one doctor says, "Why do you not have abortion?" and he says, "You should have come to me first, the doctor you went to is a kind of God, no doctor can now touch you, they will not go against him." So I have no way to get abortion. This was a miracle.

I feel bad, day and night you can see me in tears. I cry for months. I beg my sisters to bring me poison, I want to die. My sister, Mary, says she will run away and leave me, she can not see me cry all the time. Mary and Margaret sit with me every day; most of the time I am sitting with Mary.

I did not tell the man that was the baby's father that there is no way I will walk again. He spent time with me in the hospital, but he did not know I will not stand. Then one of his friends asks me, "Does he know you will never stand?" I say, "No he does not know." I tell his friend, "tell him." I got injured in July so I remember in December the man took his leave after his friend told him. I don't know what happened, he never visited me again. I feel nothing that he left, you know why? I had nothing to do with him, he can go away; I didn't get hurt that he ran away. On this day I am pregnant and I think only about my baby.

My father think it like a punishment, he say, "she pregnant, can't walk, why does this happen to my daughter?" My sister tell me this after he dies.

One day I have pain, they want to give me pain killers. I say no, I accept it, I am pregnant. I have friends that come visit me; I am very famous, so my bed was surrounded with friends all the time. Everybody comes, it so nice.

Then, it was in the morning, I have bad pain, so I tell my sister my stomach is pain. Then she says, "Ahhhh , do not worry this is because of pregnancy, everything fine, you need to have a drink, then we will go down to therapist." She knows I am in labor but does not tell me; she does not want to frighten me, but she knows what is going on. They take me to a room, I think it is for therapy, but for delivery. Someone comes in and says, "Faustina, you look ready." He tells my sister I am in labor and my sister told me, and I shout again, "Nooooo." [laughs] During the delivery there was a meeting between the doctors they want to give me drugs for pain and they want to transfer me to surgery for C-section. Other doctors say, "No, we do not need to transfer her, we will take care of her. We can deliver her." I start to cry, they say, "No Faustina, do not cry."

When I was in labor my nurses say, "I can see the head," they say, "bring forceps." Both of the people delivering me, I am listening very carefully as to what they want to do. I hear them say bring the forceps, she cannot push. I know babies delivered with forceps have many problems, their head is hurt and cannot think right. I say, "I can push." I push. They say, "Ahhh what are you doing?" I say, "I am pushing," They say, "Do it again." I do and they say, "Jesus" and I say, "Jesus." Then she is born, I start to cry and they cry with me for ten minutes. We are crying and shouting. Just after the delivery I found out it was a baby girl. But the time I was in delivery my sisters were waiting outside. Then they gave baby to me. I could feel her, I try to give her my breast. I try, she cannot eat yet, but I say, "Eat." They say, "Wait, Faustina." They smile. Then we cry again.

Then that afternoon my sister, Mary, comes to me and she pretend she open something to give me. She say, "Faustina I have brought the poison, do you want it? Now you have started a new life." A beautiful life, I had reason to live.

Then after delivery I stayed for two months in hospital; then I was discharged. When I was pregnant, during Christmas they told me to go home. I went home four days, then back and forth to get use to being at home. Then after birth they told me to go home for a few days. I said, "How can I go with my daughter?" They say, "Go." I stay with my sisters. Then doctors told me I need to go back to hospital, and I say why should I go back to the hospital? I stay at home. I was living with Rosie, my oldest sister, and other sisters all live together there to care for me.

I have no money. Mary, my strong sister, says we will sue the father for money, he has much money. We took him to court, women never do this! At first I want nothing from him, but Mary says no. We won, now he pays us. Mary says, "Now you can buy a conga." We can take care of ourselves.

KASI [Kilimanjaro Association of Spinally Injured] people come to visit me; they want me to work with them. But I tell them, I am not disabled. They say, "Faustina you need to meet people, you need to take care of yourself." Mary say, "You must do things for yourself." They tell me about KASI, you need to go with them and see what they are doing. A woman came and tell me to go to South Africa for classes. I say, "Who will watch Tunu?" My sisters say they will, they say no, you need to go. It was very difficult, I had to stop breastfeeding. I stop nursing Tunu, my family takes care of her, so I can go. I went to South Africa all alone in a plane, stayed there for two weeks, and you know what, I meet many people with spinal cord injury and I learn every day. They show me how to look pretty, to cook, to do laundry. A lot of things, how to use my wheelchair, for the first time I got this wheelchair. They taught me lots of things. All of us there were first learning. I was not alone. It changed me.

I came back to Moshi and I was smart. It was like what happens when you learn. My sisters surprised that I had changed, and meeting people with the same disability.

I was very much able to take care of my daughter. Cooking using charcoal, Tunu helps. She is very helpful to me, she goes to the shop. I remember when she was little she would go to the shop for me, she hand money to the shopkeeper and they give me what I need. I tell Tunu one day to go to shop, but do not cross street, okay, baby? Do you know what she did? The shop did not have what we wanted, so she crossed the road and came back with soda, beer. I say, "Tunu, where did you find it?" She said, "I had to go to shop across the road." I am surprised, but happy. Next day she say, "Mama, let me cross the road again." I said, "No that is highway." She say, "Mama, why you afraid? You can watch me." I say, "Go baby." She say, "Mama, you do not have to worry, I am here and God is watching over us." She can go to shop, she can go to market. I say, "Tunu my baby, the window and door must be open all the time." She says, "I will open and close it for you." She is always there to help me. As a mama I have to worry about her all the time, but she is good child.

And the most important thing making me happy is doing things with Tunu. We can do everything together. I have picture of how I did it with my mama, so I want to do same way my mama trained me. I say thank you Jesus. Working together with my daughter is my happiness. I begin to cry, I already confess to her when I accept pregnancy; I say, "God, forgive me, forgive me, I do not know what I need."

And then KASI looking for a secretary and they give me a chance and I did it. I was lucky, it very hard to say how I did it. I want to work, I need money to look after Tunu, so I applied. Working for KASI it helps improve my confidence, to talk to other women that are disabled. In 2004 I founded women's group to deal with women's issues. Women with special needs, we talk about needs and rights and a lot of things. During the training, women need help, I found out we need something special for women. When we talk about problems of disability, women have special needs.

There are 35 women members. It is important we support each other because more women die than men, a much higher number. This last year we lost two members. Most of them die with bed sores because if women married they are neglected. Marriage is punishment to them; their husbands not care for them. They don't have assistance at home, they don't drink water at home and they have no food. Other women have nowhere to go. If husband has spinal cord injury the wife cares for him.

Women with spinal cord injury do not get married, men do. They are looked at as a burden. Difficult to have a baby if injured, women are in very bad situation. I do not want to get married, I do not think about it. I have Tunu, she is my husband, my friend, my everything.

Our group meets and then we give whatever we have, if she is suffering and dying of hunger—we try to care for her. Our community helps. One woman, her children are all married, and her husband neglected her. I advised her last born to come back and talk to her husband. He did, now the husband helps more. [I then commented: I remember last time I was here there was a woman with a spinal cord injury and pregnant. People came and asked you to go talk to her. Faustina then continued:] The baby passed away. She had a very bad time, last time I went to see her was two months ago and no one came to visit her.

Tunu is going to primary boarding school, this is for her, you must have a good education. First I introduce the issue to her, she say, "Oh mama, you think I can be far from you, I use to sleep with you. I touch your breast and now you want to take me to boarding school, I miss your breast so much." I say I take her. She say, "No, you will be here alone, I will miss you, who will help you?" Then she say she will talk to school administrator. She went for interview. She said it was fine, I tell her to tell me about it so I can decide if she fail or pass. She says, "They want me to write A to Z, that is all I can remember."

This is a very good school, but she cannot make it unless we change things. She is in grade 2 in Moshi, but I told her we are going to start at grade 1 until you have learned all. She said in this school I will study hard. She likes it very much. This is the best place for her. When she was going back to school, she said, "Mama, it takes money, you pay all of this. I want to go back to this school, I want to stay there." She loves it. She is number 2 out of 35 students. I couldn't believe it.

I am 37 years old, the biggest thing I've done, that really touched me, that I'm proud of is . . . Tunu! Everyday I say it is good to be a good mother, to give her a good education, to show her that I can do it. It is my responsibility to look after her. This is what I pray to God for day and night.

CONCLUSION

Faustina lived with a dynamism that could inspire the world. When she described herself as famous, she could not have found a more fitting word. She exhibited not only courage, but joy in a life that held what some would consider insurmountable challenges. She is a storyteller, a proud mother and the secretary at Kilimanjaro Association of Spinally Injured (KASI).

KASI was started by Dr. Henry Nyamubi, a young doctor who was paralyzed in an auto accident at the age of 25. Primarily because of his status as a doctor, he benefited from health care and rehabilitation services in Europe. He is now 48 years old. He is paralyzed from the waist down and has limited use of his hands. In spite of his disability he has found the energy and passion to be the executive director of KASI, a non-governmental organization to help others afflicted.

The purpose of KASI is to provide training, education, and mobility aids for individuals with spinal cord injuries. In addition, groups like the one Faustina started for women offer emotional and physical support. KASI is also an advocate for the rights of people with disabilities. In order to encourage their recognition by the government and other organizations, research is needed on the frequency and care of individuals with spinal cord injuries. Research in general in the country is lacking, so it is not surprising that currently almost no research has been conducted on individuals with any disabilities.

DISCUSSION QUESTIONS

1. What did you admire most about Faustina?
2. What life lessons did you come away with from her story?
3. What were the most important elements in Faustina's recovery? How do they relate to creating programs that would assist other people in adjusting to a disability?
4. At one point Faustina considers suicide; discuss the ethics of letting a person choose to end their own life when faced with a physical illness or disability. Do you think this right should depend in any way on the culture and circumstances one lives in? How?

5. How did Faustina's early life help frame the person she became? How did her spinal injury further expand her character?

6. Do people with spinal cord injuries constitute a separate cultural group?

7. Could government policies help individuals with a disability? Brainstorm policies you would like to see put into place.

8. Faustina faced a combination of psychological and physical problems. Discuss how the two interacted with each other.

9. Is there a correct way to deal with grief and loss? Discuss essential elements of grieving. Is the grief process culturally bound?

10. Does Faustina's identity change as her life changes? If so, in what ways?

11. Discuss the role serving others played in Faustina's recovery.

12. When discussing her father's decision not to remarry, Faustina says his choice is motivated by a deep love for his children. What cultural aspects of marriage are revealed by this statement?

13. There are undoubtedly many differences between Faustina and yourself, at least some of them cultural. Yet there are so many aspects of Faustina's story that could be understood by women and men in countries all around the world, if there was not a language barrier. What are some of these aspects? Lessons? Morals?

14. When Faustina found out she was pregnant many people around her expressed varying opinions. Her sister told her not to have a child, her doctor told her to keep her baby. What do you think motivated these opinions? How do you think Faustina was influenced by these? Discuss the implications that the decision was largely taken out of Faustina's hands.

15. Do you understand Faustina's refusal to admit that she was disabled as a coping mechanism? Can you relate to this? Do you think it helped or hindered her progress?

16. Faustina recalls that a woman who has a spinal cord injury is unlikely to marry, and is considered a burden to a potential spouse. She then says a man with the same injury will most likely marry, and be taken care of. Discuss how gender roles in Tanzania are revealed with this double standard. How do you think this would play out in your culture?

17. When Faustina recounted her time in South Africa, she said, *They taught me lots of things. All of us there were first learning. I was not alone. It changed me.* How do you think social support and camaraderie changed Faustina's experience and, subsequently, her life? Which other women in the book, do you think, could have benefited from this kind of support group? How do you think their lives could have been different?

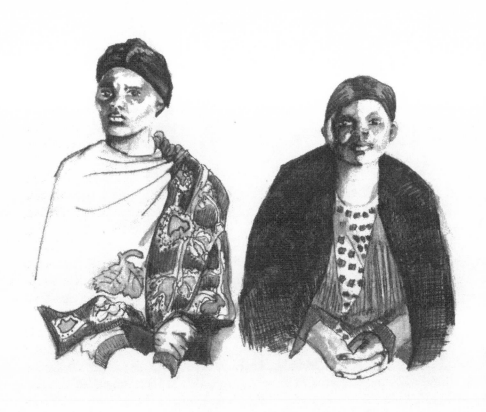

Chapter 13

Mary & Angela

Mary and Angela represent two voices among the estimated 1.4 million living with HIV/AIDS in Tanzania. Many believe this number is confounded with the problems of accurately measuring the prevalence of a virus/disease with both debilitating social stigma and taxing physical manifestations.

Both Mary and Angela made accommodations in their lives to obtain medicine for their condition. Anti-retroviral (ARV) drugs are administered throughout Tanzania at no cost. Obtaining ARVs becomes cost-prohibitive, however, when one factors in the cost of traveling to centers administering the drugs. The bus rides are often expensive, but even more expensive is the day of travel that replaces a day of work. Health practitioners are reluctant to give people drugs in large quantities because they fear that without the incentive of acquiring medicine, people might not come in for regular check-ups.

One of the major drivers of the HIV/AIDS epidemic in Tanzania is the practice of having multiple and concurrent sexual partners. This practice is common for those who are in polygamous marriages. While first wives often have a say when it comes to choosing the second wife, this is not always the case. Furthermore, sexually transmitted infection (STI) testing is not as common in Tanzania as it is in the United States, so even those wives who help choose a second or third wife are often not able to make decisions based on health status.

The issue is further complicated by the cultural practice of wife inheritance. If a man dies, it can be expected that his brothers or other male relatives inherit his wife. This is one method of ensuring that the family's physical possessions remain in the family while also providing security for the woman. Whether or not the husband died due to complications surrounding HIV/AIDS is often not known, sometimes due to biomedical constraints, but also because social stigma can discourage disclosure of health status. Wife inheritance, thus, can unknowingly extend the spread of the disease.

Most of us would agree that there is a great deal of shame that comes with an HIV/AIDS diagnosis. Mary and Angela were very brave in telling their stories, but were often censored by a conditioned proclivity for silence. When I met them, they were sitting next to each other, cloth covering every inch of their bodies except for their faces, both wearing frowns that appeared to be one step away from tears.

As you read their stories, pay particular attention to the role of shame in Mary and Angela's lives. Briefly take a moment now to consider how perceived shame might be different for public figures in the United States who are living with HIV/AIDS. How might the quality and intensity of shame involved in an HIV diagnosis be related to treatment options and availability, and subsequently, prognosis?

MARY

My name is Mary. I am 36 years old. I am a member of the Hehe tribe. I am a Christian. Both of my parents are dead.

My parents were ill when I was growing up. My mama died from tuberculosis and my Baba died from a fever. I have six sisters. We all helped out around the house when my parents were dying.

When I was 31 years old I found out that I am living with HIV. My husband has not been tested. We had seven children together. Two have died. None of them have been tested. This is the village, it is not like the city.

My husband has three wives. One has already died.

I have not told my husband about my health status. Before my doctor told me I had HIV, he told me I had tuberculosis. When I told my husband about that, he refused to support me. I don't feel like there is anything new to tell.

When I told my sisters, they asked me how I got the sickness. "What will you do?" they wanted to know.

When my sisters have money, they support me. They want me to continue to get treatment.

I feel bad that my parents are dead, instead of being here with me . . .

When I told my children, some of them cried. My son, Bitali, cried because his father was refusing to attend to his mother. My children have now accepted my condition.

Women who are living with HIV and AIDS are separated from their communities. They are not invited to talk with the neighbors. No one is educated about HIV. Some people are loving, but not to me.

I'm sorry . . . I am too shameful to tell you anything more.

ANGELA

Angela is my name. I have lived for 43 years. I do not know how many more years I will live.

Four years ago, to this day, my husband died. He had three wives. I was the second. I met him because he moved to my village to be a teacher. In Tanzania, after you become a doctor, a nurse, a teacher, or any kind of professional, the government tells you where there is a need for you and then you move to that place.

So he moved to Tulgamangane, and then we met for the first time. He told me he was unmarried. I loved him very fast, so we got married. He did not pay a bride-price because my parents were already dead.

We had three children together. My youngest child has died. He was born at a normal weight, but after about three years he stopped growing and then he died when he was eight. I cared for him all by myself because my husband died when our young son was two years old.

My husband was coughing very badly. He was suffering from diarrhea, and he was complaining that his legs were numb. When I asked, he told me he was dying because he had tuberculosis.

Before my son died, his doctors also told me that he had tuberculosis. His heart was having problems doing its work, and his legs had become paralyzed. Both my son and my husband were living with paralyzed legs before they died.

A year after my husband died, his third wife died. I decided to get on a bus, go into town, and get a test for HIV. The test came back positive.

Oh, it's a very silly story how I found out that my husband had a wife already before he married me!

One day I was preparing lunch. I heard a man and a woman outside, and then someone stuck their head inside called: *Is anyone there?* I was very happy to meet these people because they said they were from my husband's town of birth. My husband and I invited them to have lunch with us.

While I prepared our food, they all chatted outside. When our meal was prepared, we all ate together. It was only then, with a full belly, that I learned who they were.

I heard them tell my husband, "We are going to bring our daughter to you. You promised to take care of her. She is your responsibility."

My husband replied, "I have married another woman. Verona was away studying."

"We do not care. You paid a bride-price for Verona. Now you must support her."

"Yes, but after I paid the bride-price, Verona was too late getting pregnant."

"You have paid a bride-price. She is yours."

My husband turned to me, and spoke. In front of Verona's parents he gave me an order.

"Have respect for Verona. You will both have to live together now." The next day, we all moved in together.

We all lived together in harmony for a short while. Then Verona got pregnant.

"I want to live alone with my first wife," my husband told me.

They found a new house just for them and they had three children there. They stayed together in that house until he died, and then she came back to live with me.

I was so sad when I found out that my body was sick with HIV. I was so shocked, it was a great surprise to me.

The medicine for HIV is very expensive. Well, most of the medicine itself is free from this organization, but I have to pay for the bus ride into the town and back home too often; that uses all of my money. I also need someone to take care of me when I am weak. I had moved in with my uncle for a short while so he could look after me. He was living in the town. I sent my children to live with my husband's first wife during this period of time.

After my uncle died, I moved back in with my children. It was a challenge for me to move back to the village. I had one brother and he was very humiliated because of me. He asked many people to discriminate against me because I was sick with HIV. I was really wishing all of those people didn't know.

I grew sicker because of my brother. My blood pressure rose and rose and I felt very weak. My brother-in-law took care of me during this time.

There is an HIV awareness organization that called my brother in for counseling. I really don't know what they told him, but now I understand that education plays a role fighting discrimination. Since my brother has spoken with these people, he has decided to accept me. This is a great example of the power of education. We need this kind of thing very much in the villages here in Tanzania.

I think my husband gave me HIV. I don't know how he got sick with it. His third wife died recently.

I was very angry when I found out that I had HIV. This anger was directed at my husband. But this feeling didn't last very long, because you can't be angry at someone who is dead. When someone dies, all is forgiven.

Now, I just remember my husband fondly and think about how our life was good when he was alive. There was a lot of food then. We had a very good house, with a roof. I like to remember my son and my husband.

Now, I have so many problems. I have this feeling that if I was with my husband I would not be in this kind of bad position.

I still think of him. I still love him. Now, today, there is no way out. If he was here, there would be a roof. If he was here, there would be food.

CONCLUSION

Mary and Angela's stories clearly exhibit how HIV/AIDS takes a toll not only on the bodies it inhabits, but on the minds of the people who live with it. Marriage is more than a societal norm in Tanzania, it is a societal mandate. Not only do many women living with HIV/AIDS watch their husbands and co-wives die rapidly—forcing them to face their own mortality—but their disease status often diminishes their future potential for re-marriage. Because many in Tanzania often derive great value from marriage, those who live with a severed potential for remarriage often express a muted sense of purpose. The organization active in Mary and Angela's community, responsible for educating Angela's brother, is working hard to break down the walls built by public shame. Angela's story should provide reason to believe that this goal is not only worthy, but—if actualized—potentially life-changing for those implicated.

DISCUSSION QUESTIONS

1. We made a cultural faux pas in asking Angela how long she thought she would live. We found out, too late, that Tanzanian culture avoids talking about events too far in the future. (In fact, in KiSwahili, there is no real word for future. In order to express the concept one must repeat the word "badaaye," which translates to "later" several times in a row.) Angela responded to our question by saying she "did not know how long she would live." How do you think her matter-of-fact response reflects the cultural practice that encourages Tanzanians not to look too far ahead?

2. In the United States, those diagnosed with a life-threatening illness are often anxious to find out their prognosis. What do you think are the greater implications of the cultural practice of not talking about the future, when it comes to disease and disease outcomes? How do you think the act of living in the world post-diagnosis might be different in these two societies, with such different views and expectations of the future?

3. What do you think drives Americans to ask for a diagnosis? How might availability of technology and medicine influence this question? How might culturally bound notions of death and the after-life influence this question, and its implications?

4. Angela chose to describe her health status by saying her "body was sick with HIV." Why do you think she chose to say it in that way? What are the implications of her choice of words? How do you think her relationship to her disease status is revealed in the way she expressed this fact?

5. Do you agree with Angela, that you "cannot be mad at someone who is dead"? How does your answer reveal differences between your culture and Angela's?

6. Do you view Mary as culpable in relation to her disease status? What do you think is driving her shame in recounting her story? If you were infected with HIV as a result of your spouse's extramarital sexual relations, would you blame yourself?

7. Why do you think Angela expressed love for her husband, and sorrow that he was deceased, despite the fact that he infected her with HIV? How do you understand her talk of the roof—a status symbol with real utility in Tanzania—to be an idiom of distress?

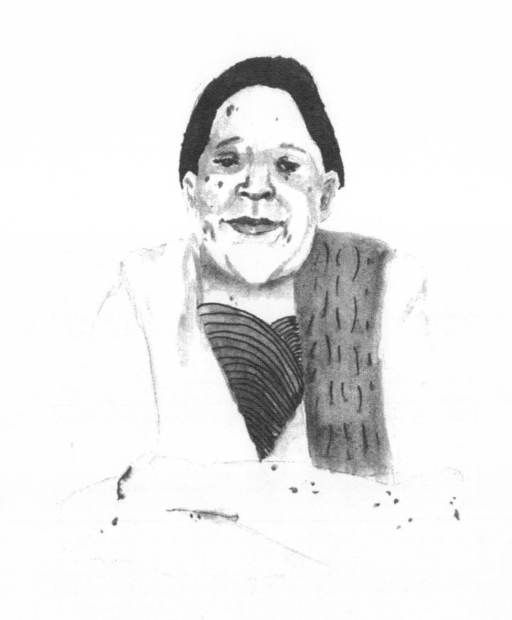

Chapter 14

Helena

There are more than 8,000 people living with albinism registered in Tanzania. At one time the sun and its skin damage were the only threats to people living with albinism, but now their lives are in danger from fellow Tanzanians. Many of these 8,000 are crippled with fear: a consequence of the belief that albino bodies hold magical—even curative—powers. Traditional healers use the skin, hair, and eyes from albino bodies as medicine, often making them rich. At least 26 people living with albinism were killed in 2008 as a result of the belief in the curative powers of albino body parts.

Despite President Kikwete's efforts to support people with albinism, the number of deaths is still rising. The president has made speeches deriding the noxious belief that is driving the killings. He even took an important step forward in publicly accepting albinos, by sponsoring an albino in parliament. Still, the public is demanding more effective methods to stop the killings, and accusing the government of turning a blind eye to the plight of people with albinism.

Helena is a woman living with albinism in the Iringa province of Tanzania. I spotted her instantly as she walked towards the house where I waited for our interview. Her skin was markedly whiter than my own, contrasting my nonchalance in applying sunscreen with the diligent effort required by her condition. As she approached the house, I could see her heavy black wig slipping around on her head, causing lines of sweat to paint shiny thin stripes on her face. When Helena dropped herself into the chair that awaited her, she did so with a huff, indicating a tired readiness to reveal the intricacies of her life.

As a result of fierce familial support Helena bears a strong self-confidence, and she does not fear for her life. She uses her interview as a political space to garner attention and support for those living with albinism in the villages.

Her humble yet brave narration illustrates the importance of social support in Tanzania for those living with a disability. Furthermore, her story draws attention to the lives of those who never experienced that support. Helena intentionally holds us accountable to think of the lives of those who were, and continue to be, prevented from reaching their full potential.

HELENA

My name is Helena Machibia and I am 38 years old. My birthday is on December 15th. Just before Christmas. My biological father left me when I was two years old, so my mama did the same. I grew up with my grandparents. My life with my grandparents was good because my grandfather was good to us. He sent us to school. He wanted us to have full lives.

I was happy in childhood but school was hard because I was told that something was not normal with me. I had no problems with my family, just with the kids at school. I remember the first time that my mother told me I was different from everyone else at school, and different from everyone in my family.

I was playing with other kids outside, and my mama ran outside to tell me that I couldn't play in the sun. I thought this was because she didn't want me out with the other kids. I was about seven at this time.

So I asked my mama, "I want to play with the other kids, why can't I play with the other kids?"

She didn't tell me in that moment. But then a few days later, my mama was walking by school and she called me outside and asked, "Where is your hat?"

I wasn't wearing my hat because, when I was with the other kids that day, I asked myself, "Why do I have to wear a hat? No one else wears a hat."

So I put it in my pocket while I was away from my mother. When we were outside, I had forgotten to put it back on my head and I walked home. Hatless.

As an older woman now, this is really a funny story. Can you imagine me, with this head, and with this skin, walking home with no protection from the sun? Thinking I would be just fine?

When I got home, my mama was mad!

"Come here and look at our arms," she said, roughly. She put our arms next to each other. "You are a different color. You cannot play in the sun because you are white. You are not my color. You must listen to my instructions."

Because of this, my mama went to my teacher and told the teacher that I cannot be in the sun.

But it was before this happened that I knew in my heart that I was white. As a young girl, there were no spots on my skin. But as I grew, I saw black dots developing. Like polka dots. I realized that this is because I was white. I said to myself, "If my mama got these spots on her skin she wouldn't be able to see them. She wouldn't know they were there. Well, only some people are white. I'm like them, and that's OK."

At school the other kids made me feel like I was white, like I was like whites, and they made me feel different. School was always very hard, also, because of my eyes. I can't see very far. The kids didn't make fun of me all the time, just sometimes. My brother was at school too, but he never spoke up for me. I don't really know why he didn't help me.

At that time, when I was a young girl, I never thought I would get married. But I've been married for 18 years now, and he's not even albino! And Eleristo doesn't have any other wives either, just one, and you're looking at her! He didn't pay a bride-price for me because he didn't have any money at that time.

We had three children together, but one of our daughters died last year from malaria. All three of my children are black, but during my births, at the last moment, right before they were born, I always wondered if they would be like me. I even hoped a little bit that they would look like me. I never told anyone that.

I thought maybe I wanted a child who was albino because I wanted to care for her properly and I knew I could. At my first pregnancy I felt fine to have a black child, I was not very surprised that she came out black. But after I pushed her out, I thought I saw a white face on my baby! I asked the nurse, "Is it a girl? Does she look like me?" The nurse told me to "hold on." I could tell she also thought maybe the girl would be like me! Then the nurse got her wrapped up and brought her over to me and asked, "Here she is, does she look like you?" I could see she was black.

All babies here come out a little whiter than they will be in real life. They are not white, exactly, but they do not have strong melanin in their skin yet, so it takes a few days before their skin adjusts and turns really black. That's why I got confused.

At my second pregnancy it was the same thing! I saw the baby, she was born without hair and she looked white! As fast as I could catch my breath I asked, "Can I see her? Can I see her?" The nurse asked me, "What are you afraid of?" She thought I was scared the baby would be white, but actually, I wanted the baby to look like me, to have the same color as me. Then the nurse told me, "Congratulations. She's not like you." I didn't really want her congratulations.

It was the same thing for the third. He was a boy, and he was not like me. And now? I will have no more babies. So there are no more chances to make an albino baby.

I don't think people treat me differently because I am albino. I feel comfortable around all people. I did talk with my husband though, a while ago, I asked him. "How do you feel to be married to me? I'm different from you." He said, "I'm ok, I don't see you as any different." It was nice to hear him say that.

In Tanzania, other people kill albinos. They believe that if you have an albino in the family it is bad luck, and that everything will go badly for you. I was already grown up when I realized this because my family was so loving. They are good Christians and they are very educated—this is why they were so good to me.

There are other false stories about albinos here. People think that if you have HIV/AIDS and you have sex with an albino, that you cure yourself. And the witch doctors think albino body parts will make them rich because they cure other diseases, so albinos are at high risk for rape and murder. This makes me afraid for my life. I have no peace. But those who are suffering are not me, they are those who are living in the village, who are children.

Because of these risks, life can be dangerous for an albino. I know a lot of other albinos here in town and I love to be around them, so I decided to become a leader for albinos. I started a group that meets once a month. There is a larger organization in the capital city for albinos, so our group is a chapter of that.

I took me two years to think about this group and decide on an aim for the group before I called our first meeting. I tried to go to offices and I got some money and I asked many people, "Do you know any albinos?" I did all of this in the town here, but there was not much I could do in the villages. Transportation is difficult here, and expensive. And I was only one person, so I could not get to the villages easily.

After two years passed, I called all the albinos, collected them in one place and told them what to do. They gave me a free room to have a meeting. I went to the broadcasting company, AM TV and told them, "I don't have any money but please, please announce that there will be a meeting for albinos in this town." They did it!

More than 20 people came! I was really happy! We all talked about the aim—to help other albinos to understand themselves. Until now, we have no office. We are still trying to find one.

We heard from the head office that we should have a vote, and I was chosen to be the chairwoman. We don't have any money, and we are still looking for a sponsor.

Our aim is to help albinos in the villages. There are a lot of albinos in the village who are born there and whose parents hide them. They don't educate them. They just see them as weak, and so they make them stay inside. I go and tell them, "You are normal. You deserve human rights." If the people we talk to are grown up, we talk directly to them. If I meet a child, I talk to their parents. I always tell grownups if it is evening outside and I have to walk home, this is fine, I will be fine. But babies can be taken by force if you cover their mouths. I heard that this is happening a lot.

Our president is an advocate for albinos. I feel very good because for a long time albinos were forgotten. We weren't known to anyone. We thank the president because this is progress—he has hired a cabinet member who is an albino. And now everyone can see this person working. He is making us known and this is good news that he is willing to elect an albino.

Life is different for albinos in a lot of ways. There are many precautions for my skin. First, I use medicated soap to kill bacteria. I also use this lotion which prevents the sun from burning. You can get it at the shop. It is available to buy, but it is very expensive. I have to buy it often, so I have to save my money to be able to afford it.

In the village, there is no access to this kind of lotion. But children are not hidden because there is no lotion. They are hidden because there is no education. With education, these things could be a lot better for them.

I can't tell you a direct story about someone in the village, but I talk with lots of people. For example, people ask me if I am a white person, or an albino, and I have to tell them that I am albino. People think, "Wow, she is so beautiful through all of her struggles." But I know that the real struggle is in the village. I want to go there and get all the albinos.

People are sometimes surprised when they see me. They call me *white person*. I hear them calling all the time, *Whitey! Whitey!* I respond back to them, "Yes, hello, how are you?" It really doesn't bother me to be called that.

I don't think if I was living in America, where the people are mostly white that there would be much of a difference in my life. The true challenge in my life is that I am serving as a mirror to others. For example, people here listen to me, they listen to what I say. Here, I am like a politician. I am a leader in the community. They all accept me. My presence is as a mirror which challenges other people to see me and then feel responsible to tell others that I am normal. That albinos are people too. That albinos can have children. This is my challenge.

But I have a question for you, too, if that's alright. Are there albinos in your country? If so, how do you recognize that they are albino??

CONCLUSION

When Helena reflected that people treat her as "a politician," she was absolutely speaking the truth. Helena's spirit could be seen from a mile away. Her presence spilled light onto the walls of the dark kitchen where our interview was held for three hours. Helena laughed often and earnestly, even when recounting traumatic stories from her childhood. Her love of life was a dominant illustration of resiliency, illustrating the effects of education and social support on the lives of those living with chronic illness and disability. We left the interview certain that Helena's passion would continue to motivate her actions every day and in every opportunity her life presented her with.

DISCUSSION QUESTIONS

1. What do you think Helena meant when she said that the aim of her organization, which took her two years to articulate, was to "help albinos to understand themselves"? Why do you think that was her aim?

2. Why do you think Helena described herself as "a mirror in the community"?

3. Helena's question at the end (*Are there albinos in your country? If so, how do you recognize that they are albino?*) serves as a reminder that her experience living with albinism in a country that is populated by a majority of people with black skin, is markedly different than the experience for a person living with albinism in the United States. How do you think it might be different? Do you think the challenges involved would be the same? Different?

4. What was your first response to the way Helena described her experience obtaining and utilizing sunscreen?

5. How do you think Helena's life would have been different if she was a man?

6. Helena spoke with diligent candor in describing her feelings about the skin color of her children. Were you taken aback when she said she hoped her children would also have albinism? Could you relate to her sentiment? How did it make you feel to be privy to thoughts she had that she had not even shared with her husband?

7. Helena never thought she would get married, yet she married someone who claims color-blindness when he looks at her. Do you think the characteristics of a strong woman possessed by Helena—self-confidence, passion, pro-activity—are regarded as attractive cross-culturally? Is the value placed on these characteristics in any way bound by culture?

Bibliography

Clark, Mary Marshall. "Resisting Attrition in Stories of Trauma," *Narrative*, 13, (2005): 294–298.

Charon, Rita. *Narrative Medicine. Honoring the Stories of Illness.* New York: Oxford University Press, 2006.

Davis, Ken. "Kill That Cripple." *Mouth Magazine Free Hand Press,* Washington, DC.1995. www.normemma.com/areut_killcrip.htm (September 25, 2008).

Eide, Arne, H., Loeb, and Mitch, E. "Data and Statistics on Disabilities in Developing Countries." *Disability Knowledge and Research,* 2005, disabilitykar.net/research/thematic_stats.html (September 7, 2008).

Egnew, Thomas, R. "The Meaning Of Healing: Transcending Suffering," *Annals of Family Medicine,* 3 (2005): 255–262.

Farmer, Paul. "Pathologies of Power. An Anthropology of Structural Violence Current Anthropology," *University of California Press,* 45, no. 3 (June 2004).

Hadley, Craig, et al. "Food insecurity, stressful life events and symptoms of anxiety and depression in East Africa: evidence from the Gilgel Gibe Growth and Development Study," *Journal of Epidemiology & Community Health,* 62, no. 11 (2008): 980–986.

Hershey, Laura. "Tanzania: Research Explores Lives of Disabled Women and Girls. Disability world." Presented at Society for Disability Studies conference in Winnipeg, Canada. 2001, www.disabilityworld.org/09-10_01/women/tanzania.shtml (February 12, 2008).

Kapuya, Juma, A. "National Policy on Disabilities, Ministry of Labour, Youth Development and Sports." *Republic of Tanzania,* 2004, www.tanzania.go.tz/pdf/NATIONAL%20POLICY%20ON%20DISABILITY.pdf (March 20, 2008).

Kereto, David, O. *Disabled Rehabilitation Program.* Maasai Evangelistic Association, Kenya. 2007, www.maasaimissions.org/projects2007.html (May 14, 2008).

Kleinman, Arthur. *Patients and Healers in the Context of Culture.* Berkeley: University of California Press, 1981.

Kleinman, Arthur. *The Illness Narratives.* Basic Books, 1988.

Kleinman, Arthur. *Writing at the Margin: Discourse Between Anthropology and Medicine.* Berkeley: University of California Press, 1995.

Kleinman, Arthur, Das, Veena and Lock, Margaret. *Social Suffering.* Berkeley, CA: University of California Press, 1997.

LCCB (Local Community Competence Building). *Strategy papers: HIV and AIDS Prevention in Tanzania and Zambia.* Arusha, Tanzania: ELCT. 2006.

Maasai Association, *Maasai People* (n.d.), www.maasai-association.com (September 15, 2007).

Mandesi, Gideon, K. Presented in seminar on Publish Sensitization and Awareness Center on Disabled Issues and Problems. Held at Msimbazi Comments Center Dar es Salaam, Tanzania. (August 27–28, 1997).

Ministry of Education and Culture. *The United Republic of Tanzania Guidelines for Implementing HIV/AIDS and Life-Skills Education Programme in Schools.* (2004), www.moe.go.tz/ (April 10, 2008).

Ministry of Health. *The United Republic of Tanzania.* 2007. www.moh.go.tz/ (March 15, 2008). Mkude, Daniel, Cooksey, Brian, and Levey, Lisbeth. *Higher Education in Tanzania.* Oxford: James Currey, Ltd. 2003.

National Bureau of Statistics Dar es Salaam, Tanzania, United Republic of Tanzania, "Tanzania: DHS, 2004 Final Report," 2005. www.measuredhs.com/pubs/pub_details.cfm?ID=566 (March 10, 2009).

Orbinski, James. *An Imperfect Offering.* New York: Random House, 2008.

Pellico, Linda Honan. Narrative Criticism. "A Systematic Approach to the Analysis of Story," *Journal of Holistic Nursing,* 25. no. 1 (2007): 58–65.

Portelli, Alessandro. "'The Time of My Life': Functions of Time in Oral History." In *The Death of Luigi Trastulli and Other Stories: Form and Meaning in Oral History.* Albany: State University of New York, 1991. First published in *International Oral History Journal* 3.3 (Fall 1981): 162–180.

Scheper-Hughes, Nancy. "The Primacy of the Ethical: Propositions for a Militant Anthropology," *Current Anthropology,* 36, no. 3 (Jun. 1995): 409–440.

Scheper-Hughes, Nancy. *Death Without Weeping: The Violence of Everyday Life in Brazil.* Berkeley: University of California, 1992.

Scheper-Hughes, Nancy and Lock, Margaret L. "Speaking 'Truth' to Illness: Metaphors, Reification, and a Pedagogy for Patients," *Medical Anthropology Quarterly,* 17, no. 5 (Nov. 1986): 137–140.

Schiller, Nina Glick, "Aids and the Social Body," *Social Science and Medicine* 39, no. 7 (1992): 991–1003.

Thomson, Joseph. *Through Maasailand: Through the Central African Lakes and Back.* (reprinted) Blue Ridge Summit, PA: Rowman and Littlefield, 1885.

Index